IDIOPATHIC SCOLIOSIS: CONSERVATIVE TREATMENT with ELASTIC BANDS

Theoretical-practical Manual of the Rovatti Method®

Emanuele Rovatti - Marco Rovatti

IDIOPATHIC SCOLIOSIS: CONSERVATIVE TREATMENT with ELASTIC BANDS

Theoretical-practical Manual of the Rovatti Method®

edi·ermes

Idiopathic Scoliosis: Conservative Treatment with Elastic Bands
Theoretical-practical Manual of the Rovatti Method®
by Emanuele Rovatti and Marco Rovatti

ISBN 978-88-7051-516-9 – Print edition

ISBN 978-88-7051-517-6 – Digital edition

A book is the final product of a very specific series of operations that requires numerous verifications of text and images.
It is nearly impossible to publish a book without errors.
We would thank all of those who communicate to us the presence of any errors found.
For instructions or suggestions regarding this book, please use the following address:
Public relations - Edi.Ermes srl - Viale Enrico Forlanini, 65 - 20134 Milan (Italy)
Phone +39.02.70.21.121 - Fax +39.02.70.21.12.83

Images: Shutterstock©™ archive (7)
Rovatti Plan® archive

Printed in November 2017 by Faenza Printing Industries SpA
for Edi.Ermes srl - Viale Enrico Forlanini, 65 - 20134 Milan (Italy)
http://www.ediermes.com - Phone +39.02.70.21.121 - Fax +39.02.70.21.12.83

Presentation

When Emanuele Rovatti gave me a draft of this manual and I was finally able to read its contents, I suddenly recalled the many events, work experiences, and stages of the long path we had traversed together, beginning almost 25 years ago with our common interest in vertebral dysmorphisms and pathologies.

I owe it to Emanuele Rovatti that, in addition to being an orthopedic specialist (in the early eighties I frequented the scoliosis department of the Gaetano Pini Institute, run by professor Giuseppe Antonio Frassi with help from the legendary professor Paolo Sibilla), I have succeeded as a physiatrist in developing a scoliosis treatment that goes "beyond" clinical progressive observation, the prescription of an orthopedic corset, correction with plaster casts on Cotrel beds, and which particularly goes beyond surgery.

Working together with him, my method of evaluating and implementing treatment for dysmorphisms has been enriched by the kinesiological experience of Emanuele Rovatti: with personalized work programs, the patients become "their own doctor", an expression dear to me for its implication of one's gaining consciousness of one's own body scheme and the symptoms of scoliosis so as to permit the patients to seek correction of their own posture.

Finally, self-correcting: this is a process of learning that allows patients to take advantage of their own potential during the growing phase or to stabilize at bone maturity.

This manual is the sum of years of practice and observation of generations of patients. In it, we can see the enthusiasm that still today drives Emanuele Rovatti, who seeks to use new methods and technical means. Enthusiasm and diligence also drive his son Marco, who is attentive, meticulous, willing to relate and learn, always ready to stimulate us with questions and ideas, and who is destined to improve in the near future with his great youthful capability and desire to understand and communicate with young and old patients.

Thus I salute the friend with whom I have shared so many work and family experiences.

Melegnano (MI), October 20, 2013

Antonio Giandomenico
Orthopedc Specialist and Specialist
in Physical Medicine and Rehabilitation
Ospedale di Circolo di Melegnano (MI)

Acknowledgements

I thank my family, which is everything to me – my wife Grazia, an unsurpassed advisor, my son Marco, and my daughter Francesca – my collaborators and my entire team.

Particular thanks to Dr. Antonio Giandomenico, physiatrist and orthopedic specialist, friend and colleague of my therapeutic team; and to Dr. Paolo Viganò, orthopedic specialist, both of whom have given me the chance, since 1989, to develop the methodology presented herein through working with a consistent number of patients.

Particular thanks also to all of the patients who, over the years, have helped us with their collaboration to put this methodology into practice.

Thanks to Lucrezia and Desirè, the models used in these pages, and to Federica Delucchi, who patiently curated the final revision of the book.

Thanks, finally, to Raffaele Grandi at Edi.Ermes, who believed in this work and promoted its publication.

Emanuele Rovatti

Preface

I have felt the need to treat "scoliosis" starting from my first experiences with the world of corrective exercise and the associated specific work programs to be performed in gyms. Then, to learn more about it, I brought my patients to Paolo Sibilla, orthopedic specialist and "great master" to whom much is owed in regards to the understanding of this pathology: he, after many of these meetings, coined the term *Rovatti's Days* for those periods of work-study and visits with my students.

I remember extremely long and intense days, which sometimes stretched on with academic discussions until two in the morning. On these encounters, he visited and I sought to learn as much as possible about the various methods, approaches to patients, and the problems therewith. He, who was in contact with our colleague René Perdriolle to whom the intuition of the three-dimensionality of the scoliotic curve is credited, shared studies, results, thoughts, and the principles of Lyon exercise. All of this has contributed to my professional growth.

During these long days (of study for me), Sibilla little by little introduced me to the vast and developing world of scoliosis and idiopathic scoliosis. By the end of the seventies, he was speaking about concepts that are now widespread but were not then, such as "posture", "awareness", "body scheme", and "centers of balance". He had already reached a clear understanding that the problem he faced could not be considered simply in biomechanical terms, as was normal in that time, but required a holistic-type approach that could evaluate the persons in their entirety, evaluating additional points of view. I also followed him when he spoke of electrical stimulation for scoliosis and his final intuitions on how to treat it. He was a great learning resource who increased and won over my interest in this pathology, and above all gave me insight into how to approach it and treat it.

This text is a distillation of the work done over more than forty years of professional activity: it seeks to offer a practical contribution via the application of a specific method of treatment. In recent years, my professional activity has been enthusiastically followed up by my son Marco. He has brought, and continues to bring, his own contributions to the specific sector of kinesiotherapeutic treatment of scoliosis: verifying, updating, and constantly improving the exercises prescribed for our patients.

This method, now a registered trademark bearing the Rovatti name, may be applied by the various professional figures who already deal with the treatment of different forms of scoliosis.

The wish is that the Rovatti Method® be widespread and known as much as possible, and above all that the culture forming its basis – that is, this type of conservative approach with the innovative use of elastic bands, which we present in this book – be disseminated.

Emanuele Rovatti

Biography

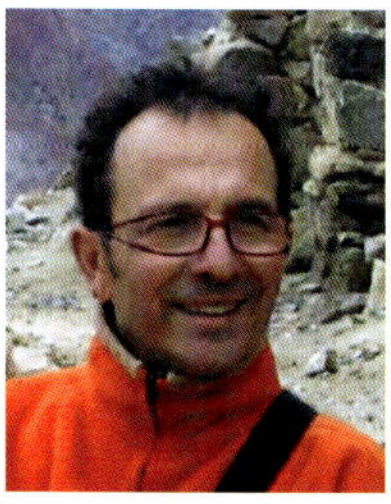

Emanuele Rovatti was born in Cavezzo, in the province of Modena, Italy, on April 17, 1949. He completed his studies with his ISEF diploma, obtained at the Università degli Studi di Milano in 1973. From 1970 to 1990, he held the role of Physical Education instructor at several secondary schools in Milan.
In 2001 and 2002, he obtained his diploma of specialization in Kinesiology and Rehabilitative Kinesiology at the School of Medicine and Surgery of the Università di Chieti, and in 2003 earned a degree in Movement Science at the same university.
From 1978 to 1994, he was the regional technical assistant for the Lombardy region of the Italian Federation of Light Athletics.
From 1986 to 2006, he was the Head of Medical Exercise and Functional Recovery at the Erre Medical-kinesiological Center in Inzago (Milan), and from 1989 to 2008 he held the post of technical Director of the "MEDI Care Center" of Melzo (Milan), kinesiology and physiotherapy department, for which company he was also the commercial head of the Occupational Medicine sector from 1994 to 2008. Since 2008, he has managed two Rovatti Plan® centers, in Melzo and in Cassano d'Adda.
Emanuele Rovatti is also a trainer in districts and schools in Milan regarding adolescent idiopathic scoliosis; he is the instructor of company courses (*ex lege 626/94, Italian law regarding safety training in the workplace)* for the "Proper movement of loads and posture" and "Skeletal risks in VDT".
He is a certified professional (clinical kinesiologist) and has made verifications for insurance companies and law firms as a kinesiological and ergonomics expert; he has performed the role of training tutor for graduate students in Movement Science and Physical Therapy.
He is associated with professional organizations such as the Unione Nazionale Chinesiologi (UNC), Società Italiana di Ergonomia (SIE), Gruppo di Studio Scoliosi (GSS), Società Italiana di Ginnastica Medica (SIGM), *Groupe Européen Kinésithérapique Travail Scoliose* (GEKTS), Collegio Toscano Periti Esperti Consulenti.
He has been dedicated to corrective gymnastics from the beginning of his professional activity. He was the student of Professor Sergio Pivetta, from whom he learned the ability to perform an exercise beginning with good kinesiological and biomechanical knowledge; he is interested primarily in the kinesiotherapeutic treatment of scoliosis.

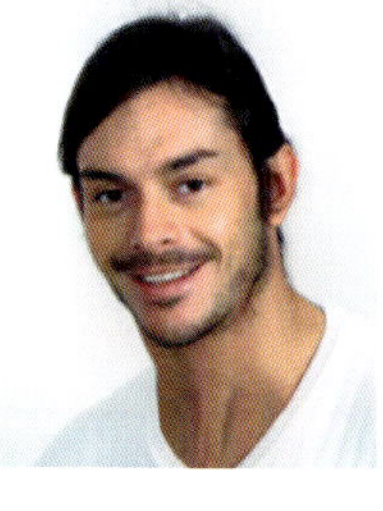

Marco Rovatti was born in Melzo (Milan) on January 7, 1982. He received a degree in Sport and Movement Sciences at the State University of Milan in October of 2007. He later received a diploma in Massage Physical Therapy.
While already in his professional training, following in his father's path, he became interested in pathologies of the vertebral column while working at the Rovatti Plan® Centers, where he had occasion to meet many professional figures and distinguished persons in the fields of both preventative and rehabilitative-corrective movement.
He is a certified ART® (*Active Release Techniques®*) therapist for the *Upper Extremity; Lower Extremity, Spine, Long Nerve Entrapment, Active Palpation, Masters Certified*. He is also FMS (*Functional Movement Systems*), SFMA (*Selective Functional Movement Assessment*), TPI (*Titleist Performance Institute*), OTZ (*"one to zero" – Health Education Systems*), and SRM (*Stress Relief Method*) certified.
He is the head of the Physiotherapy sector of the Rovatti Plan® Centers.
He attends the SOMA Osteopathy Institute of Milan.

to Paolo Sibilla
who showed me the path

to my wife Grazia and to my family
who have always supported me in following it

to Niccolò, Jacopo, Enea, Andrea, Mathias, and Emma,
children of my daughter Francesca, my beloved grandchildren.
May I be able to see them grow and develop the enthusiasm
and the passion that have always distinguished my professional activity

Table of Contents

FIRST PART

Scoliosis: From Postural Examination to Conservative Treatment

SECOND PART

Treatment with Elastic Bands: Specific Work Programs

Introduction

With this book, our intention is to bring particular attention to the treatment of several problems relating to scoliotic pathologies. The topic of scoliosis will not be dealt with directly, as that would be redundant in some way. The following (also Italian) Authors have exhaustively analyzed the topic: Paolo Sibilla, Stefano Negrini, Vincenzo Pirola, and Sergio Pivetta, to cite those closest to us; there are many others as well. We, in fact, refer to their studies and publications for all scientific analyses on the topic.

Instead, in these pages, we would like to provide basic information in order to introduce our personal contribution to the treatment of these pathologies. In fact, the data emerged from the statistical analyses of the progress of the pathologies in these cases, representing over forty years of work, are very encouraging, just as the results produced by the methodology implemented and experimented by now on hundreds of patients are very satisfying.

This book is aimed, thus, at the "insiders" and those who are interested in the problem of scoliosis. It could be used both by young colleagues in need of materials to consult and by patients well-prepared by their own therapists, so as to become a stimulating tool for working at home as well, on a personal path of growth and awareness regarding the topic of their own posture.

At a convention in Milan in 1974, we had already begun to speak of this method with a contribution titled "The use of elastic bands in the treatment of idiopathic scoliosis". Today, given the progress of the methods and new knowledge regarding this pathology, many further developments have taken place. Over almost forty years of work, the method, which is now registered as the Rovatti Method®, has been widely used, following the clinical evolution of many cases for many years. A series of specific work programs has been honed, constantly verified, perfected, and personalized for each case.

Boys and girls, young and adults have been treated; in some cases it was possible to follow personal growth over time for many, many years. In some cases, we were able to observe two generations of the same family. The passion for this work, together with the results obtained, have always been, and still are, the incentive for continuing in this direction, to refine the working method.

We believe that there may still be many additional starting points to expand upon with regards to conservative treatment and the study of scoliosis, and we hope that this material may be the basis for our young colleagues' continued work according to this vision.

FIRST PART

Scoliosis: From Postural Examination to Conservative Treatment

1

Scoliosis and Kinesiotherapy

Kinesiotherapy uses the techniques of movement; the therapist makes use of these and all related assistive techniques, such as massage, active or passive mobilization, medical exercise, therapeutic sports, treatment techniques with mechanical devices, and functional exercises.

Kinesiotherapy is successfully applied in pathologies of the spine, particularly in idiopathic scoliosis in all of the different states of severity: from scoliotic attitude or deviation with favorable prognosis, to structural scoliosis of a progressive type that is non-reducible (including pre- and post-cast treatments or surgery), and painful adult scoliosis. It is naturally indicated in all phases of correction with an orthopedic corset.

Kinesiotherapy always has a fundamental role in the long task of postural correction and rehabilitation, whether it is the only therapeutic recommendation or it is used in strict collaboration with an orthopedic specialist and surgeon.

The objectives sought in kinesiotherapeutic treatment of scoliosis are the correction or the containment of the progression of the curve, the improvement of the spinal support structures, the improvement of neuro-motor control, the aesthetic improvement, the containment of psychological damage, the postural rehabilitation and the reduction of pain, with an increased awareness of one's own body.

The therapist has the fundamental task, via regular and repeated evaluations, of collecting and providing all of the objective data necessary for the observation of any progression of the scoliotic curve, always in collaboration with a therapeutic team.

In all cases described above – and generally in all cases of scoliotic pathology – the methodology of three-dimensional correction with the use of elastic bands is indicated. To become aware of one's own posture, reactions, and corrections so that one may then progressively refine and internalize the new correct body scheme: this is, in extremely brief summary, the objective of the specific work programs of the Rovatti Method®.

1.1 SCOLIOTIC ATTITUDE AND SCOLIOSIS

First, we must make an overall distinction between scoliotic attitude (or paramorphism) and true, structural scoliosis (or dysmorphism) (figure 1.1).

Scoliotic attitude (paramorphism) is a deviation of the vertebral column only on the frontal plane; it involves no rotation. This is almost never a source of concern, except for some rare cases. Preventative kinesiological treatment and diversified sports give optimal results in these cases.

True scoliosis (dysmorphism) implies, on the contrary, a deviation of the spinal column on all three spatial planes: *frontal*, *sagittal (lateral)* and *transverse*.

The *sagittal* or *laterolateral* plane is involved in a reduction of physiological kyphosis; the *frontal* plane is involved in lateral curvature. Additionally, the vertebrae on the side of convexity (normally) rotate on the longitudinal

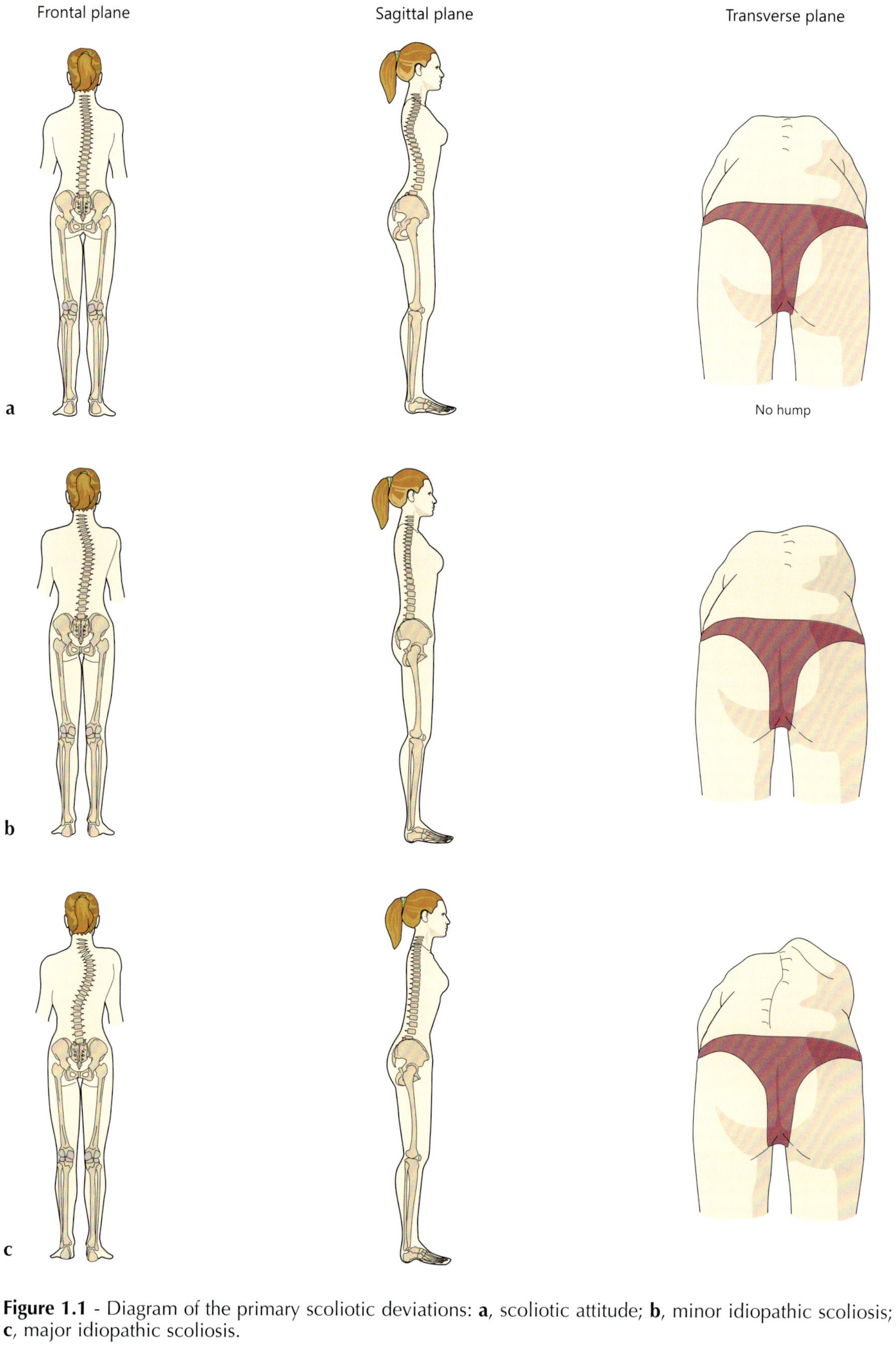

Figure 1.1 - Diagram of the primary scoliotic deviations: **a**, scoliotic attitude; **b**, minor idiopathic scoliosis; **c**, major idiopathic scoliosis.

axis, creating the characteristic "hump" (rotation on the transverse plane). Scoliosis is essentially a three-dimensional deviation of the vertebral column:

- lordosis on the sagittal plane;
- lateral curvature on the frontal plane;
- rotation on the transverse plane.

It has been widely noted that scoliosis evolves with physiological growth and maturity, worsening during the period of greatest pubertal development: normally before, during, and after menarche for females and at the same time as the change of voice and other signs of secondary pubertal maturity for males. The greatest risk of evolution of the curve is shown with Risser (skeletal maturity indicator) 0/1+, 1+, and 2+.

It is exactly in this delicate phase of development that kinesiotherapeutic and orthopedic devices must be used strategically and precisely. Puberty, in fact, is characterized by significant growth both in terms of stature and weight, as well as by a hormonal shift: all factors predisposing one to the rapid aggravation of scoliosis. This happens independently of the causes that provoked it. For the majority of cases, the cause of the deviation from the physiological skeletal curve is unknown – thus one speaks of **idiopathic scoliosis**.

> This chapter of the book attributes several quotations and ideas to certain Authors and Colleagues (names are indicated in parentheses). These acknowledge collaborations, comparisons, and discussions that the Authors would like to keep track of independently of their publication in subsequent writings, as they are fundamental to the definition of the method of kinesiotherapeutic treatment described further.

1.2 CLASSIFICATION OF SCOLIOSIS

The literature presents many ways of classifying scoliosis and deformities of the spine. There is one type of classification that essentially considers the **causes of the pathology's onset**, dividing scoliosis into: a functional and reversible type; a structural, non-reversible type; and the idiopathic type, meaning that it is not possible to attribute a specific cause to its onset (this constitutes the greatest number of cases). There also exists a traditional form of classification that subdivides idiopathic scoliosis according to the **curve type**: combined (or double) scoliosis, and single-curve scoliosis, which is in turn subdivided into dorsal and lumbar. In modern terms, many Authors (recognized within the *Gruppo Studio Scoliosi*) have described curves as "**primary**" and "**secondary**". Scoliosis may also be classified according to the **angular measurement** of the curve: an objective measurement in degrees according to Cobb's method. Other Authors prefer classification by **age at onset** (infant scoliosis, youth scoliosis, adolescent scoliosis, adult scoliosis). Let us also recognize, for the sake of completeness, the possibility for classification according to recommended treatment, a classification that begins from the objective measurement of the degrees of curvature of the spinal column and subdivides scoliosis substantially into three classes: that for which periodic orthopedic oversight and kinesiotherapy are recommended, that which requires orthopedic aid and kinesiotherapy, and finally that which requires strict medical monitoring, a cast corset, and possibly corrective surgery.

These classifications are universally accepted and shared, and are often made reference to within this book. However, the primary classification system used in this book is the most modern one, which considers these spinal pathologies **from the perspective of the associated risk of progression** of the scoliotic curve(s) (figure 1.2).

- Group A: minor scoliosis or paramorphism;
- Group B: structural scoliosis or dysmorphism;
- Group C: severe dysmorphism;
- Group D: dysmorphism at full skeletal development.

The choice of this classification is related to the construction of the rehabilitative protocols proposed by the Rovatti Method® and illustrated further in the book.

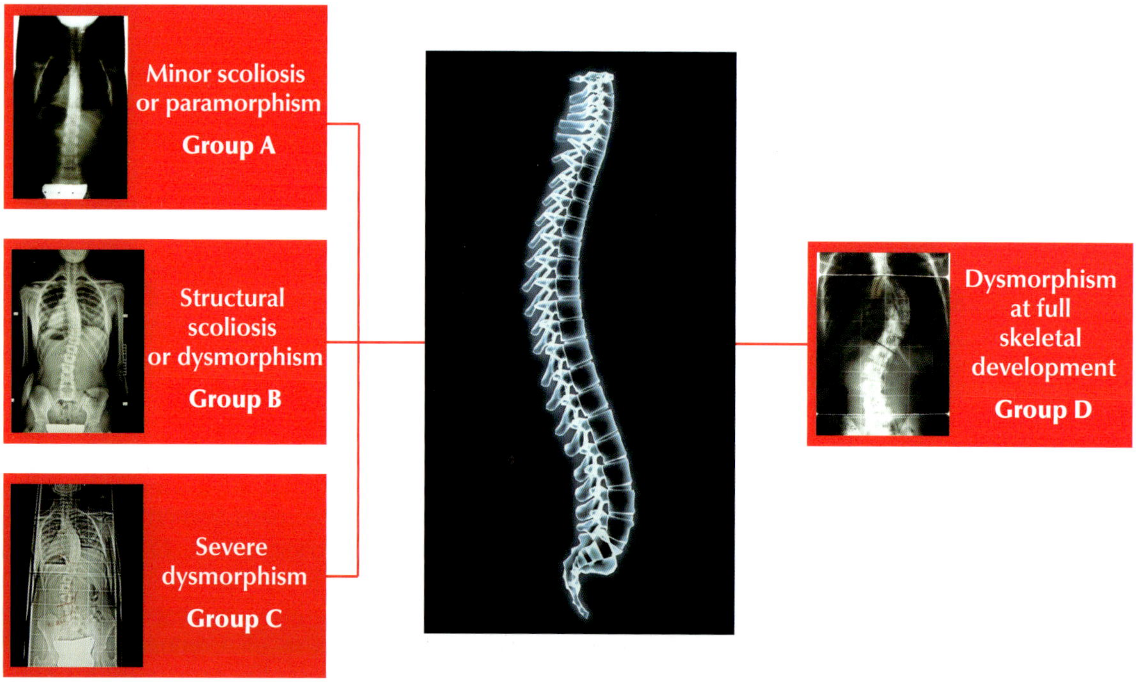

Figure 1.2 - The classification of types of scoliosis based on the risk of progression of the scoliotic curve is at the base of the Rovatti Method®.

1.2.1 Minor Scoliosis or Paramorphism

Normally, scoliosis in which a hump of less than 5 mm and angle of torsion less than 5 degrees is found upon kinesiological examination is considered **minor scoliosis**.

Paramorphism generally involves no rotation on the transverse plane.

Many of these cases involve subjects of young ages. In patients under 10 years of age, it is still useless to seek the formation of an "awareness of the deformity", because the processes of cortical maturation are still not sufficiently devel-

---

Adolescent Scoliosis

Scoliosis is idiopathic in 90% of cases. Idiopathic scoliosis is a symptom of a complex syndrome that involves different functions of the body (Sibilla). Among the causes that have been hypothesized, the most realistic is the alteration of body scheme, vestibular function, and spatial perception; that is, it is correlated with a proprioceptive disorder. In such cases of proprioceptive disorder, the deformation of the column is the natural response for reestablishing muscular balance (Sibilla).

When the curves change physiological normality on the sagittal plane (kyphotizing or flattening), the spine responds on the frontal plane by compensating in those areas rendered most mechanically weak on the laterolateral plane (Lyon method).

A varied work protocol and the search for a good aesthetic aspect may contribute to greater psychological motivation and thus more active participation of young patients. Kinesiotherapy (medical exercise or vertebral kinesiology), with the preparation of a personalized plan, is proposed as an excellent means of obtaining satisfying results.

---

oped. With these young patients, a recreational-athletic path is recommended to refine coordination and motor abilities. Only later, if the indicator parameters suggest a worsening of the condition, will a rehabilitative approach be implemented. These subjects must be monitored semiannually for preventative purposes.

Recalling the Authors of reference on the subject of idiopathic scoliosis, we remind readers that the predictive elements that determine scoliotic progression are the type of the curve, the patient's birth age and bone age, the patient's sex, and the severity of the curve (Sibilla). The first pubescent signs mark the beginning of the period in which progress of the scoliotic curve is at its maximum (Dimeglio). Normally, 30 degrees is a critical value for a scoliotic curve, beyond which scoliosis worsens if the subject is growing and of prepubescent age (Perdriolle).

Regarding **paramorphism** (and so-called "scoliotic attitude"), we remind the reader that good or bad posture is directly proportional to the interaction between the skeletal system, muscular system, spinal centers, upper centers, and, therefore, to the balance of the sensory systems (Sibilla). For this reason, proprioceptive work is always recommended, as both exteroceptive stimulation (sight, hearing, skin receptors) and proprioceptive stimulation (joint, tendinous, muscular receptors) can cause proper postural adjustments in scoliosis patients, which will become automatic if repeated continuously (Cristofanilli, Sibilla).

Figure 1.3 shows a diagram of the organization of movement via the sensory-perceptive capability.

It is good to remember that kinesiotherapy does not have the goal of correcting scoliosis, but that of teaching the patients a series of proper behaviors that are useful for their own pathological situation; behaviors that, with time, should be understood, internalized, and become automatic responses (Stagnara; Mollon; De Maurey; Negrini, 1992). "**It is not exercise that corrects, but the patient who corrects himself!**"

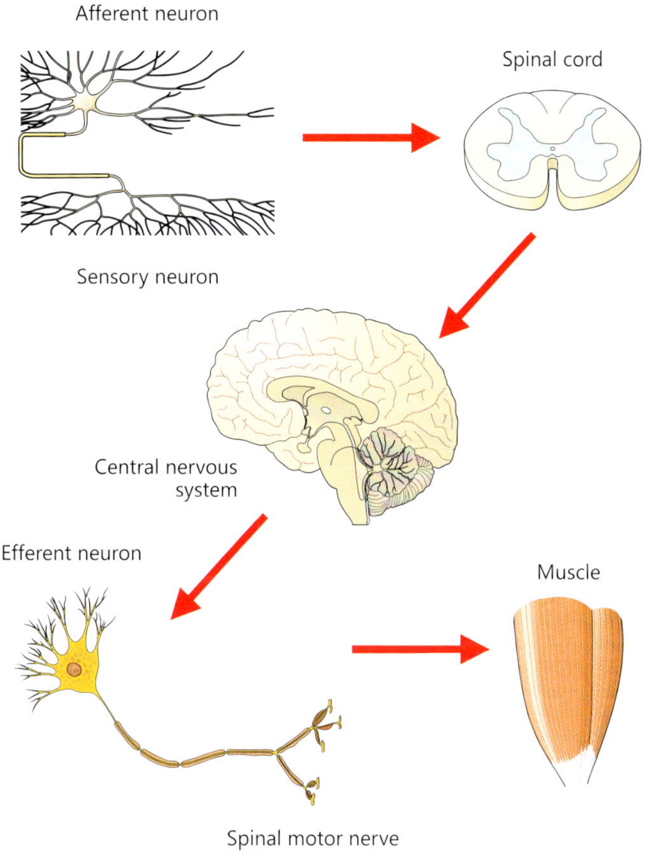

Figure 1.3 - Organization of movement via sensory-perceptive capability (Sibilla, 1998).

Therapeutic Approach

For the treatment of scoliosis, it would be proper to have a therapeutic team made up of various professionals who can guarantee a complete approach and a multidisciplinary view of the same problem. The team should be composed of an orthopedic physician and a physiatrist, a kinesiologist and/or a physiotherapist, and possibly also a psychologist specialized in problems linked to spinal pathologies, a gnathologist (postural problems linked to dental malocclusion), an osteopath, and an orthopedic technician (for purposes linked to insoles and corsets). If adolescents and children are to be treated, it is appropriate that operations be coordinated so as to involve the parents and possibly the trainer (if the subject practices sports). General practitioners, though not included in the therapeutic team in a strict sense, have the task of coordinating and monitoring therapeutic progress.

Treatments

In minor scoliosis, treatments should involve mobilization of parts of the body only if necessary, but not near the principal scoliotic curve (which is more likely to develop further if mobilized). On the other hand, it is appropriate to work on muscular strengthening, the development of equilibrium reactions, and thus on the improvement of coordination.

Kinesiotherapy for paramorphism is important due to its influence on anti-gravitational muscular strength and its ability to improve neuromuscular abilities. Sport is the active version of kinesiotherapy, as has been affirmed by the exponents of the *Gruppo Studio Scoliosi* (GSS). Thus, for postural paramorphism, kinesiotherapy associated with sports is recommended.

Lastly, but certainly not least importantly, particular attention should be paid to respiratory education.

$R = n^2 + 1$

a, straight column:	$0^2 + 1 = 1$	(R = 1)
b, column with one curve:	$1^2 + 1 = 2$	(R = 2)
c, column with two curves:	$2^2 + 1 = 5$	(R = 5)
d, column with three curves:	$3^2 + 1 = 10$	(R = 10)

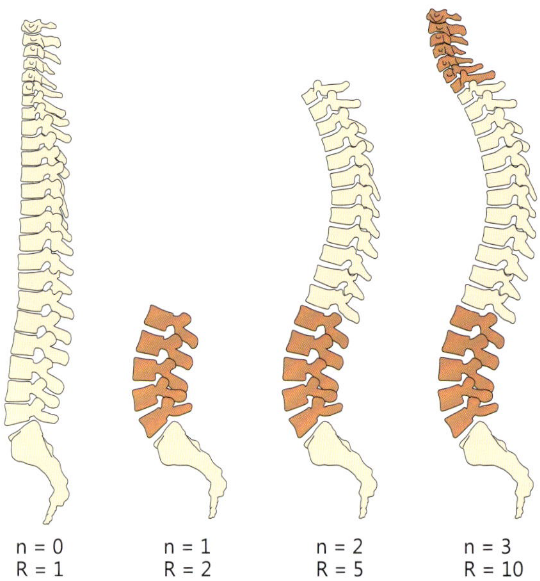

Figure 1.4 - The spine resistance to load, according to Kapandij, is proportional to the square of the number of curves plus one.

1.2.2 Structural Scoliosis or Dysmorphism

As for paramorphism, it is proper to have a therapeutic team in the treatment of structural scoliosis and dysmorphism (Group B).

There are four physiological curves: **cervical lordosis**, **dorsal kyphosis**, **lumbar lordosis,** and **sacral kyphosis**. When these are reduced in number, the spinal column is more subject to weakness. The most severe cases of scoliosis are those that accompany a marked dorsal flatness, as greater pressure is exerted on the spine on the frontal plane due to the fact that the curves on the sagittal plane are reduced (Sibilla).

Figure 1.4 illustrates the importance of maintaining the physiological curves on the laterolateral plane; these are used to support gravitational load. The presence of curves increases the spine's resistance to compresson.

Compression forces (loads and gravitational forces) on the vertebral column in orthostasis exert – both perpendicularly and laterally – loads on the vertebrae and discs (decomposition according to the parallelogram of forces).

The vertebra inclination causes these forces to induce a forward or backward slippage of the directly underlying vertebra, increasing or reducing its reference curve.

Consequently, the **spine resistance to load** is correlated to the number of curves (n), observed on the sagittal plane, as pointed out by Kapandij. In particular, Kapandij correlates the spine resistance (R) to the square of the number of curves (n) plus one:

$$\mathbf{R = n^2 + 1}$$

To describe the column resistance, we can also consider the **Delmas Index** (I), which is the ratio between the height of the column (H, measured on the sagittal plane, from the plate of the first sacral vertebra to the atlas) and the length of the extended column, that is the column deprived of the physiological curves (L). The value must be multiplied by 100:

$$\mathbf{I = H \times 100/L}$$

The index physiological value is approximately 95 (physiological limits between 94 and 96).

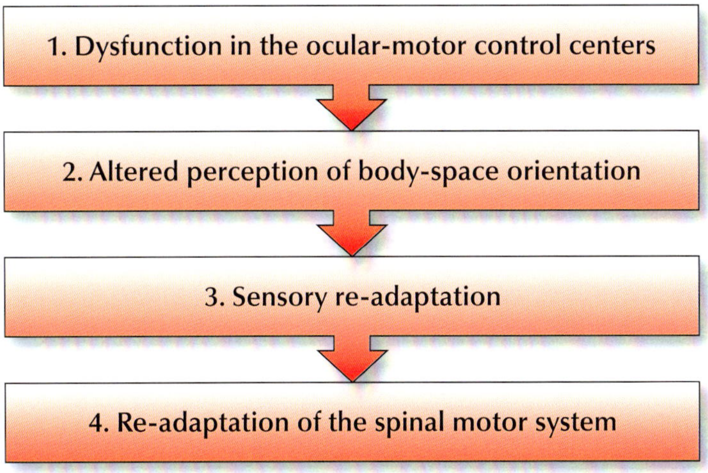

Figure 1.5 - Compensation in idiopathic scoliosis (Sibilla).

The disadvantage of this approach is that the evaluation to obtain the Delmas index can only be performed on the anatomical part.

Delmas thus demonstrated that a vertebral column with pronounced curves is dynamic functional, while a column with less pronounced curves (or without one/more curves) is static functional.

Therapeutic approach

The treatment of the most severe cases of scoliosis (namely those with flat, elevated dorsum) generally excludes extensor exercises, as they increase both the degrees of the curve and specific vertebral rotation.

With progressive structural scoliosis, corrective extensor exercises may be performed, but with particular attention paid to the recovery of normal sagittal curves. In this case, it will be the therapist's ability that will allow for the comprehension of the subject's type and the evaluation of when and where to implement these exercises. The mobility/rigidity of the curves, muscular tone/trophism, and the subject's kinesthetic sensitization must be periodically evaluated in order to adapt the therapeutic protocol.

Patients with diagnoses of structural scoliosis or vertebral dysmorphism often have prescriptions for corrective orthopedic corsets. With these patients, a personal therapeutic protocol must be established, comprising awareness exercises, proprioceptive exercises, respiratory exercises, aerobic capacity strengthening exercises, and corrective exercises performed in a corset.

Currently, the most used orthopedic corsets are the "modified Lyon", which is ideal for double scoliosis; the "La Padula", prescribed for lumbar scoliosis; the "Chenêau", for double scoliosis; the "Sforzesco", and the "Milwaukee". With this latter, a therapeutic protocol should be established that includes kyphotizing exercises, trophicizing exercises in a corset, and proprioceptive exercises. Additionally, particular attention should be paid to respiratory education. Recently, this Milwaukee corset (a corrective girdle that tends to flatten the sagittal kyphotic curve) is used for kyphosis in adolescents or children.

Though patients with minor scoliosis require breathing exercises, both for the ribs and the diaphragm, more severe cases must also include respiratory exercises that incorporate shaping: that is, exercises in which an attempt is made at reshaping the trunk towards its correct form. Isometric exercises are also useful for the paravertebral muscles in order to work on their position-holding capabilities.

Asymmetrical movements with scoliosis should be performed on the basis of overall improvement, without creating new tensions or false straightening (Lyon method). The objective of the treatment is to reach, in the post-corset phase, a new postural model via the reorganization of one's own movements in

Table 1.1 Kinesiotherapeutic Rehabilitation Protocols

Kinesiotherapy upon removal of cast corset and introduction to orthopedic corset
Awareness of the correction made
Coordinative ability development
Perception of proprioceptive and exteroceptive stimulation
General exercises
Notions of ergonomics
Moderate sports activity
Exercises of the group "structural scoliosis or dysmorphism"
Kinesiotherapy in the post-surgical phase
Carefully avoid exercises that prematurely stress the operated area
Pelvic and scapulohumeral girdle mobilization exercises
Respiratory exercises (to favor exhalation)
Perception of proprioceptive and exteroceptive stimulation
Ergonomic work to favor spontaneity of movements
Moderate physical activity
Stretching to reduce any muscular tension

space and time (Viel). According to Sibilla, compensation for idiopathic scoliosis may be achieved by following the progression indicated in figure 1.5, a diagram that should be attentively considered for corrective protocols.

Treating structural scoliosis, exhalation work should be given priority for a more shaping effect. Too much focus on inhalation may lead to deformation of the thorax in cases of significant rotation, since the intercostal muscles increase rotation (Lyon exercise). The objective of kinesiotherapy in these cases is to create a proprioceptive "natural corset" (Stagnara).

The more motor experiences one has, the more the motor abilities are increased. Motor ability is the result of learning, and becomes automatic with repetition.

1.2.3 Severe Dysmorphism

Cases of structural scoliosis that reach 40/50 degrees, a limit representing a clear index of progression of the curvature, belong to group C. This is true even after the skeleton reaches Risser 5+ (Lyon school), which denotes full skeletal development. Patients with this type of scoliosis must generally be treated with surgery. It has been shown that good pre-operation physical preparation with a specific protocol helps thc success of the therapeutic path taken. In the pre-surgical phase, exercises of a preparatory type must be arranged with the patient: mobilization exercises may be carried out before the orthopedic or surgical treatment in order to recover greater mobility. In the postsurgical phase, without a corset, the patient will perform overall physical activity as well as stretching exercises to reduce muscular tension, balance-rhythm-dexterity-coordination exercises, and upper and lower limb strengthening exercises, taking care to avoid working on the arthrodesized area.

When the patient wears a cast, work of general trophism is recommended: corrective asymmetrical exercises, exercises of the extensors, and exercises of the exhalation muscles in derotated conditions. Additionally, exercises must be done to improve the patient's maximum aerobic capacity. The objective, during the months of cast-based correction, is to create a good muscular framework. We remind the reader that vertebral instability is associated with less strength in the trunk muscles.

Table 1.1 shows, in summary, the key points of two recommended kinesiotherapeutic rehabilitation protocols: severe dysmorphism upon the removal of the corset, and in the phase immediately following surgery.

1.2.4 Dysmorphism at Full Skeletal Development

The last group of scoliosis types (Group D) for which the kinesiotherapeutic application via the use of elastic bands is useful regards adults: namely, dysmorphism at full skeletal development.

In painful adult scoliosis, the kinesiological protocol involves stretching, cervical/dorsal

Lyon Exercise

"It is not exercise that corrects, but the patient who corrects himself" – this is the premise and the essential point of implementation of the Lyon method, the school born from the meeting of various orthopedic specialists, physiatrists, and physiotherapists in France at the *Centre Médico-Chirurgical des Massues* of Lyon. These experts, starting around the second half of the 1950s, carried out significant research work as a team and became a standard-bearer in the sector of scoliosis studies. Among them, we particularly remember Stagnara, de Mauroy, Charrière, Mollon, Ollier, and Perdriolle, whose contributions on the three-dimensionality of the scoliotic curve and the dorsal spine's tendency to become lordotic in cases of idiopathic scoliosis are fundamental to the modern approach to the kinesiotherapeutic treatment of scoliosis. The Rovatti Method® itself is derived from the Lyon school, and begins from exactly these basic concepts in order to propose its new methods with the use of elastic bands for "rehabilitating" and "shaping" the spine in search of corrections on the three spatial planes. The elastic bands – as if they were the therapist's hands – teach the patient to perceive, internalize, and self-correct.

The *Centre des Massues* in Lyon has become well-renowned in the interim among professionals working with scoliosis and researchers of spinal pathologies. Many Italian professionals have received theoretical and practical instruction there.

Among the most interesting theoretical fundamentals forming the basis of the Lyon method, which is always in search of new kinesiotherapeutic, surgical and orthopedic methods and methods regarding the definition of clinical evaluations, is the principle of not rejecting scientific evidence coming from other schools of thought.

The work of Stagnara, an orthopedic surgeon, was fundamental to the construction of an approach that worked on balance and thus to the planning of non-mechanical neuromotor rehabilitation (subjects with scoliosis have problems with balance). The construction of the school's method started from this point, which seeks correct posture via the stimulation and refinement of balance reactions. Finally, for the subject (who must learn to correct him- or herself, and who must be the protagonist of his or her own rehabilitative pathway), the awareness is fundamental. For this purpose, the recording of objective data, their comparison over time, and the awareness not only of defects and deformities of the spine but of one's own corrective trajectory and new body scheme, sought via the prolonged holding of correct postures, are extremely important. Active partecipation in the exercise protocol is required, and sharing with the patient the results, reached via exercise and documented by the objective data collected, is recommended.

pulling, reshaping and correction of humps, trophism of the upper and lower limbs, and general motor activity.

In approaching the topic of painful adult scoliosis, it must be kept in mind that this often involves subjects with osteoporosis or osteopenia. The rational and focused kinesiotherapeutic approach should necessarily consider several objectives in these cases:

- respect of particularly at-risk areas;
- use of greatest aerobic capacity;
- muscular reinforcement, preferably of an isometric type;
- gradual, personalized, constant motor activity (evaluate the subject's abilities attentively, considering age and sex).

Particular attention should be paid to mobilization exercises: mobilization exercises of the spine are generally contraindicated because greater flexibility may favor worsening of the scoliotic curve over time. For antalgic purposes, mobility is useful for joints outside of the spine, which act as a release from endogenous and exogenous demands placed on the vertebral column.

2

Postural-functional Kinesiological Examination

A proper postural and functional kinesiological examination is the basis of the proposed kinesiological treatment, and is indispensable in screening to identify the patient's vertebral problem and how it should be treated. It consists of an analytical and possibly comparative examination to gather useful information for the creation of the individual treatment plan. The collection of objective data allows to compare the results and values found with postural control examinations. Postural reevaluation (kinesiological examination) should be made regularly throughout the course of the corrective treatment, perhaps approximately every six months.

For each patient or case treated, it is necessary to prepare a **personal sheet** on which to write and subsequently compare all of the possible data regarding the patient clinical history and their therapeutic and corrective path.

The kinesiological examination is organized into different phases with a sequence of measurements and tests administered to patients:
- postural kinesiological examination;
- functional kinesiological examination.

The first part of the evaluation, the **postural kinesiological examination**, focuses attentively on the static-dynamic morphology of the patient in different positions (figure 2.1): a frontal examination (anterior-posterior; figure 2.2), a lateral examination (laterolateral), frontal and dorsal observation, first anterior and then lateral observation in anterior bending of the trunk (Adam's test), and teleradiographic image in orthostatic position.

The second part of the evaluation, the **functional kinesiological examination**, focuses on muscular tone-trophism and joint mobility, and is the basis for defining the personalized rehabilitative protocol.

The kinesiologist's tools for properly carrying out the postural and functional examinations are varied and include: lifts for the evaluation of any dysmetria in the limbs or pelvis, a digital camera, a goniometer, a plumb bob, a rigid measuring stick and a flexible extendible measuring tape for circumference measurements, dermographic pens or markers, a scoliometer, a humpmeter, and a Cobbmeter affixed to the backlit board for reading x-rays (figure 2.3). In the kinesiologist's office, finally we must not leave out the kyphometer and the podoscope for morphological evaluation.

2.1 PERSONAL SHEET

During the kinesiological exam, the professional compiles a personal sheet for each patient, which will show all pertinent data while following the corrective path taken so as to chart the patient's progress. The personal sheet, accompanied by images, must report the following information:
- full scoliotic history and familiarity up to the date of the exam under way;
- patient's personal data;
- annotations of x-ray data;

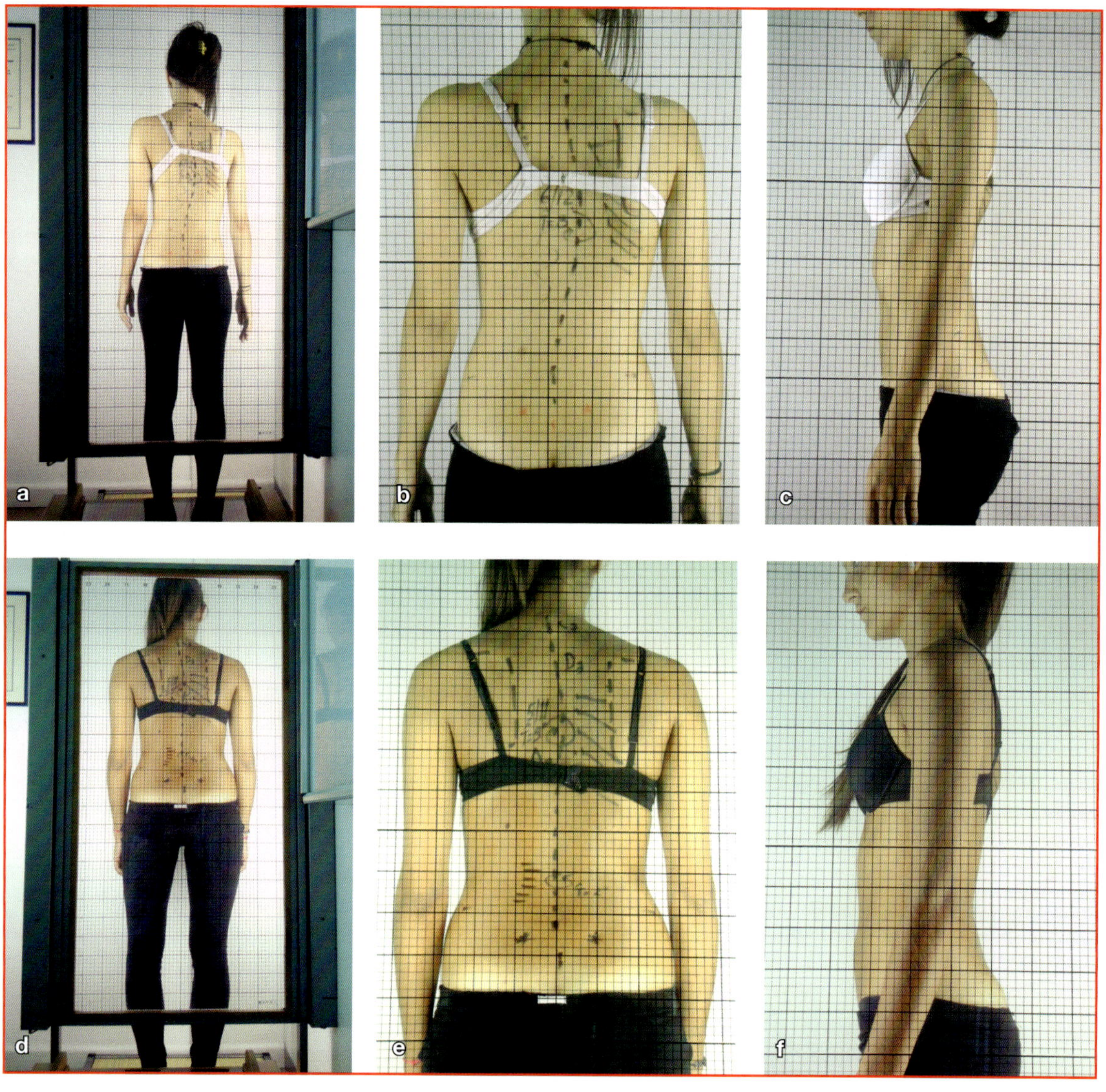

Figure 2.1 - Postural examination in two different subjects who show different degrees of scoliosis. In orthostatic position, with the help of the kyphometer, the assessment of the frontal profile (**b**, **e**) and of the sagittal or lateral profile (**c**, **f**). The evaluation of the aesthetic profile, which is to be compared semiannually, has a strong psychological and motivational impact, above all for juvenile and adolescent patients.

- static-dynamic morphological data;
- photographic evaluation;
- recommendations for the personalized work program.

Today, modern technologies (computer devices and dedicated applications) allow for a much simpler and immediate creation of images and cataloging of the various phases than ever before, and thus may be more accessible for the patients themselves.

2.2 POSTURAL KINESIOLOGICAL EXAMINATION

After accurately collecting on the personal sheet the patient's personal and family information for kinesiotherapeutic evaluation, the kinesiologist, before proceeding to the series of evaluations included in the examination, must properly highlight all landmark points in order to facilitate objective instrumental measurement. The kinesiologist performs this with

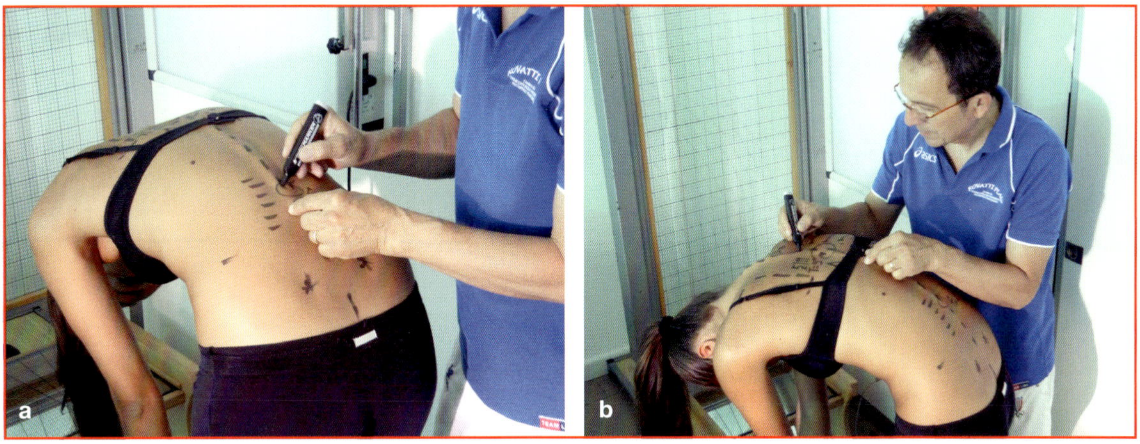

Figure 2.2 - Frontal morphological examination: measurement of the spinal apophyses and humps. All of the landmark points are highlighted for the objective measurements. Marking of spinal apophyses (**a**) and humps (**b**).

the help of a dermographic pen or a simple marker. In the figures, the same evaluations are shown on two different subjects with different degrees of scoliosis.

2.2.1 Symmetry of the Shoulders and Scapulae

This evaluation is performed by having the patient assume a proper posture, in orthostatic position. The frontal posterior view, with inked landmark points to facilitate reading, shows the symmetry or possible asymmetry of the shoulders and the scapulae. The kinesiologist attentively evaluates both the upper and lower profiles of the scapulae (figure 2.4).

2.2.2 Waist Triangle

The waist triangle is the space formed by the inner profile of the arm and the contour of the hip flank. In cases of dorsolumbar scoliosis,

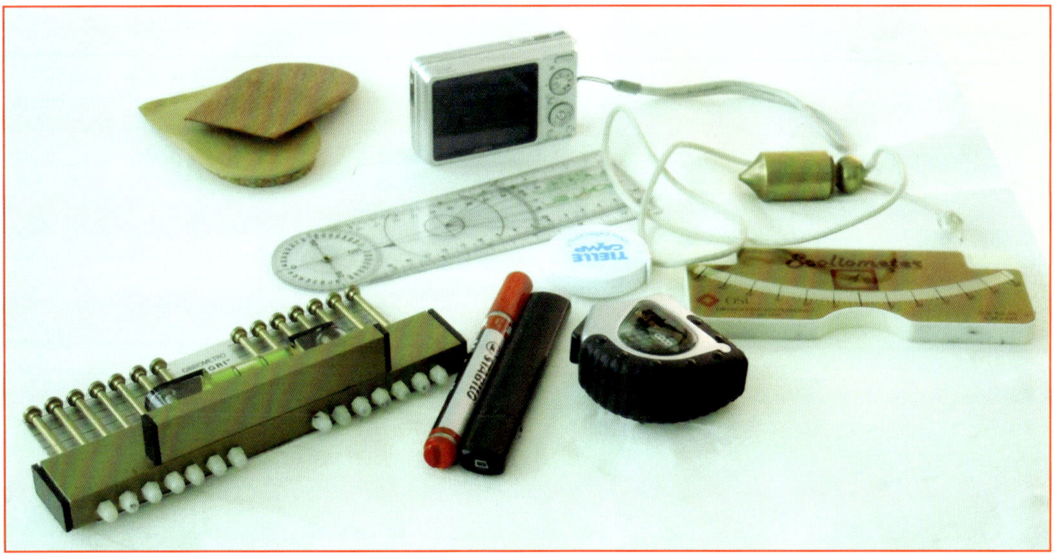

Figure 2.3 - The instruments of the postural kinesiological examination. Clockwise: lifts for the evaluation of dysmetria in the lower limbs and pelvis, digital camera, goniometer, plumb bob, scoliometer, measuring stick, extendable measuring tape (circumferential measurements), markers, humpmeter. The Cobbmeter applied to the backlit board for the reading of x-rays is added to these.

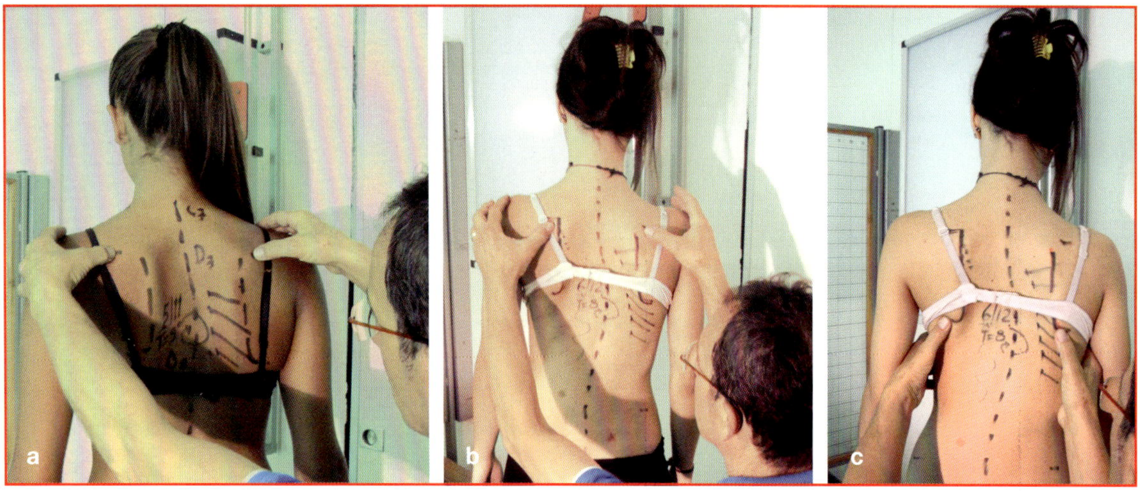

Figure 2.4 - Postural kinesiological examination, frontal morphological assessment: symmetry of the scapulae and shoulders, upper profile (**a**, **b**) and lower profile (**c**).

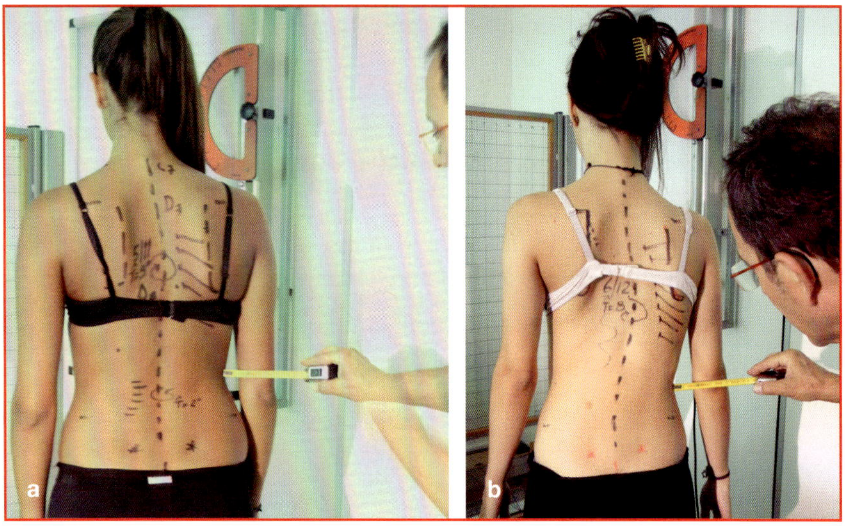

Figure 2.5 - Postural kinesiological examination, frontal morphological assessment: measurement of the waist triangle.

the progressive movement of the side entails the reduction and deformation of the waist triangle, a sign of the existence or worsening of scoliosis. Measurement is taken with the rigid extendable measuring device, with the patient in orthostatic position, from the posterior frontal view (figure 2.5).

2.2.3 Occipital Axis

The examination evaluates any overhang of the occipital axis, assessed with the plumb bob. The alignment between the occipital protuberance and the intergluteal line must be evaluated. Normally, the plumb bob must be positioned at the center of the line. A deviation on the left or right may reveal scoliosis (figure 2.6).

The balanced occipital axis, on the contrary, is a factor of a favorable prognosis for the correction of scoliosis.

2.2.4 Anomalies Aaffecting Other Parts of the Body

The complete morphological examination must consider any anomalies in other parts of the body, particularly the thorax, the knees, the feet, the temporomandibular joint, and any associated problems of dental occlusion (figure 2.7). The evaluation of plantar support is done with the use of the podoscope (figure 2.8).

2.2.5 Analysis of Sagittal Curves

The analysis of the curves of the spine on the sagittal plane is of extreme importance. Measurement is done in orthostatic position, with evaluation on the lateral (laterolateral) plane made with a plumb bob and a rigid measuring device (figure 2.9). Below, the three appropriate measuring points are indicated:

- C7 (maximum convexity);
- T12;
- L4 (maximum concavity).

Figure 2.10 shows the physiological parameters of the curves on the sagittal plane.

2.2.6 Balance of the Pelvis

With the patient in orthostatic position, the balance of the pelvis must be attentively evaluated to show any existing dysmetria.

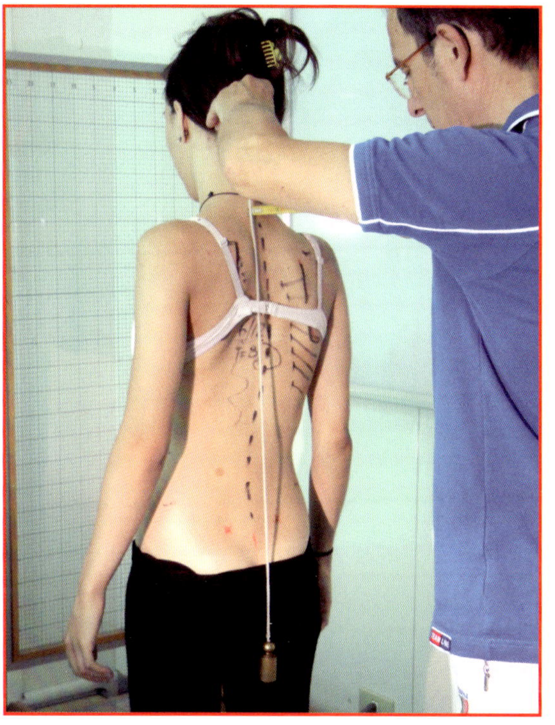

Figure 2.6 - Postural kinesiological examination, frontal morphological assessment: measurement of overhang of the vertebral column at C7.

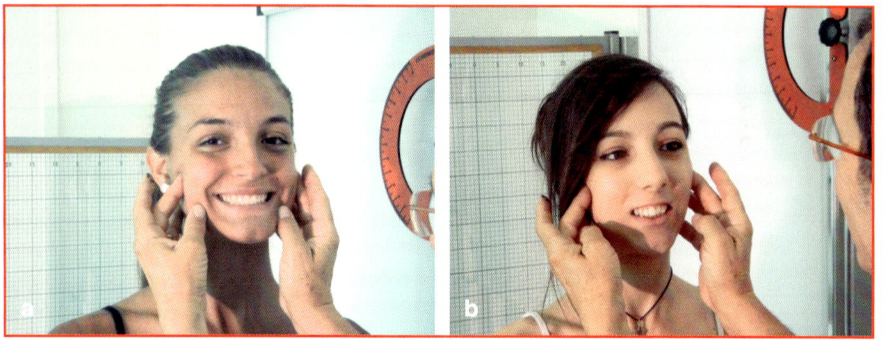

Figure 2.7 - Frontal examination: assessment of dental occlusion.

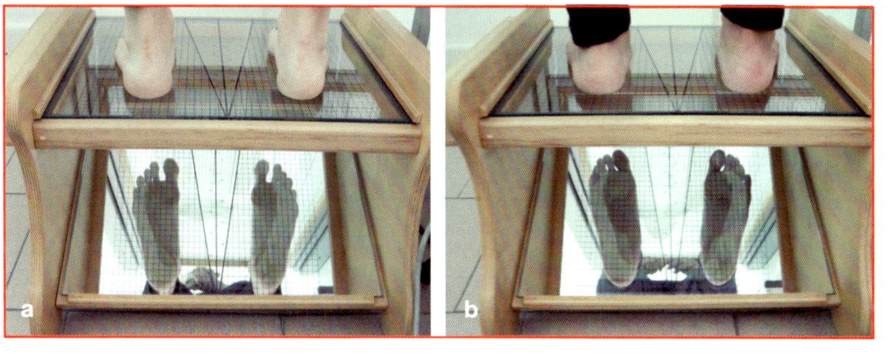

Figure 2.8 - Frontal examination: assessment of plantar support with podoscope.

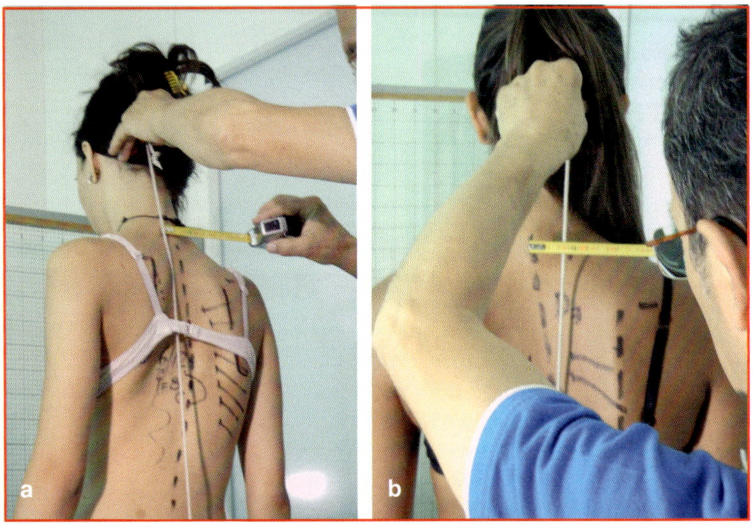

Figure 2.9 - Postural/lateral kinesiological examination: measurement of kyphosis at C7 (measurement also repeated at T12).

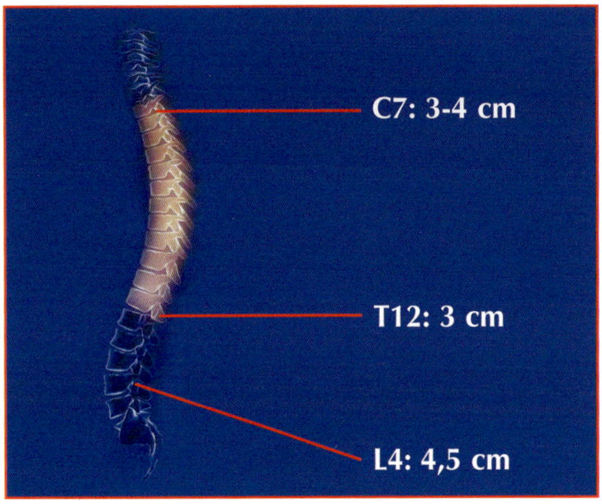

Figure 2.10 - Physiological parameters of the curves on the sagittal plane.

The landmark points are the iliac crests (figure 2.11). The evaluation is performed with anterior and posterior frontal view:

- anterior superior iliac spines (ASIS);
- posterior superior iliac spines (PSIS).

2.2.7 Measurement of Humps

The evaluation and measurement of humps, respectively the dorsal and lumbar hump, are performed in the anterior bending position (bending test or Adam's test). The bending test consists of anterior bending of the trunk, performed while keeping the lower limbs stretched, which allows for the evaluation of the extent of a hump or humps. The measure-

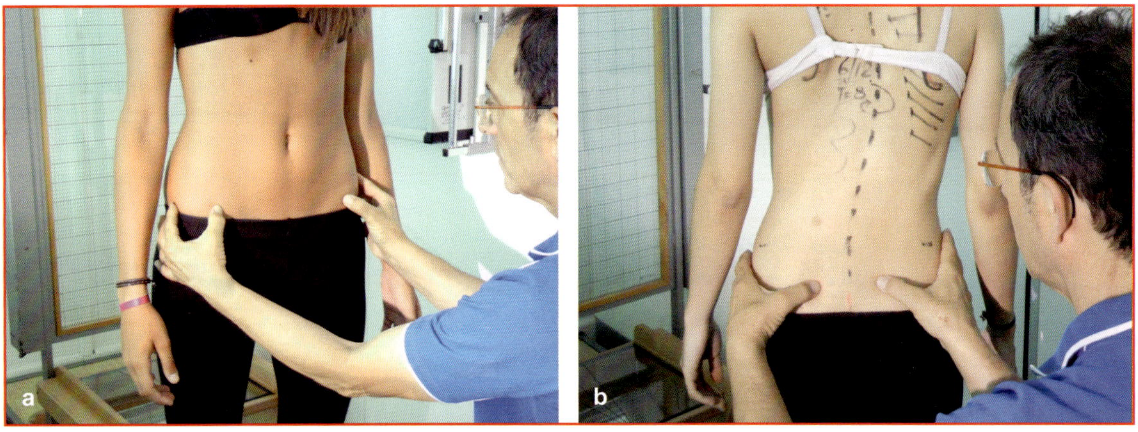

Figure 2.11 - Balance of the pelvis: assessment from the anterior superior iliac spines (ASIS, **a**) and from the posterior superior iliac spines (PSIS, **b**).

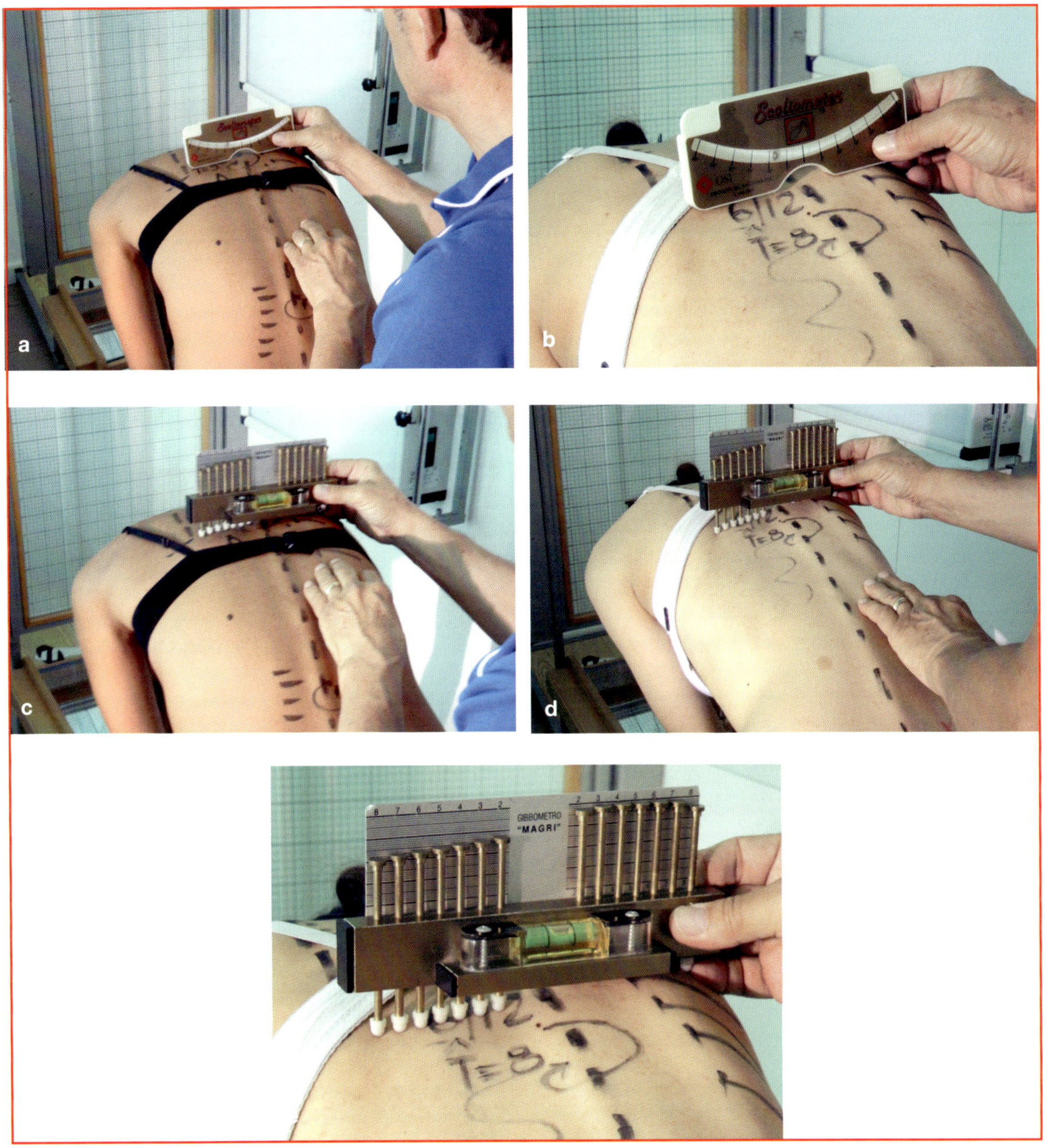

Figure 2.12 - Postural kinesiological examination with anterior bending. **a**, **b**, Measurement of the degree of torsion of the apical vertebra with a Scoliometer® (reading in degrees); **c**, **d**, measurement of the dorsal right hump with the Magri humpmeter (reading in millimeters); **e**, enlarged view of the instrument.

ment is performed with two instruments: the scoliometer and the humpmeter, and is repeated for all humps (figure 2.12).

The scoliometer (Scoliometer®) gives an objective measurement of the degree of torsion of the apical vertebra, read in degrees.

The Magri humpmeter evaluates the height of the hump in millimeters.

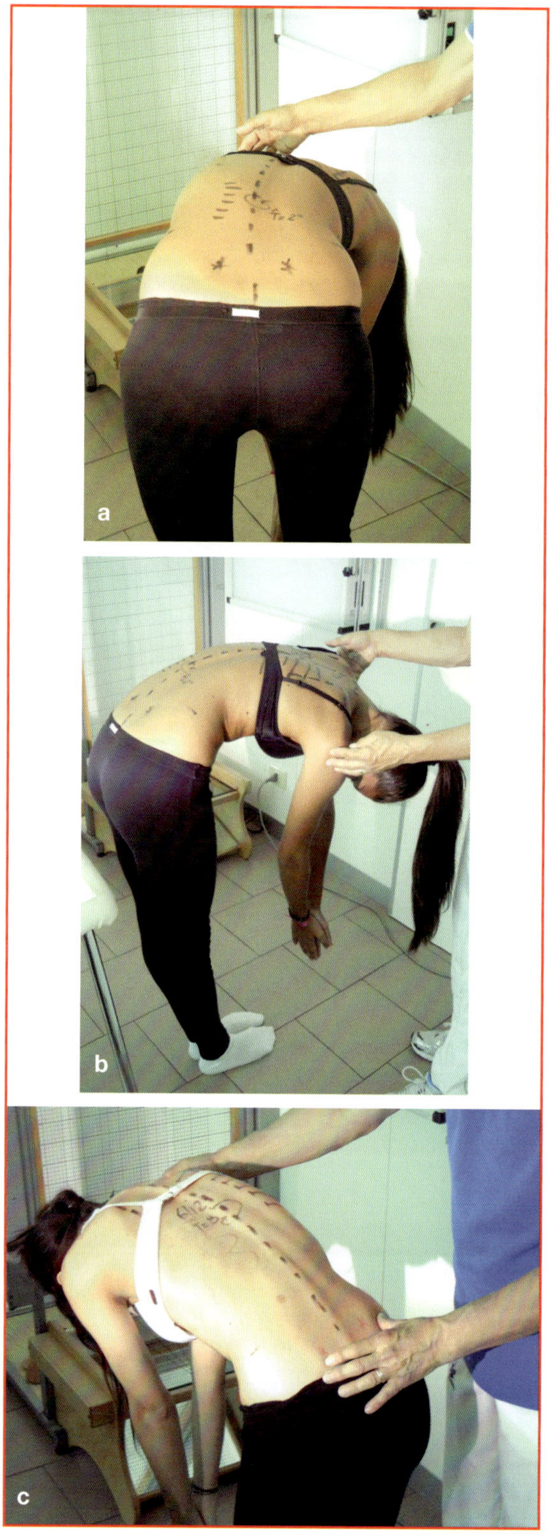

Figure 2.13 - Evaluation in lateral bending position for the verification of the reducibility of the scoliotic curve (**a**); right lateral view (**b**) and left lateral view (**c**).

2.2.8 Evaluation of Reducibility of Scoliotic Curves

The patient holds the anterior bending position, as in the previous evaluation, and then slowly moves into the lateral bending position by moving the trunk alternately to the right and left (figure 2.13). This allows evaluation of the reducibility of the scoliotic curve, according to defined parameters:

- + complete reducibility;
- ± incomplete reducibility;
- – non-reducibility.

The + sign indicates the so-called "inverted hump" during lateral bending, and is a sign of a favorable prognosis (non-structural scoliosis). The ± sign indicates an intermediate case, evidenced by the disappearance of the hump during lateral bending. Finally, the – sign indicates the non-reducibility of the curve in a case of structural scoliosis (unfavorable prognosis) (figure 2.14).

2.2.9 Teleradiographic Evaluation in Orthostasis

The frontal x-ray evaluation in orthostasis allows assessment of the degree of rotation of the vertebral peduncles, which in cases of scoliosis range from the physiological condition (both normally visible) to a progressively pathological condition, until becoming fully hidden (figure 2.15).

- 0 on axis (physiological condition);
- 1+;
- 2+;
- 3+;
- 4+ the peduncle is fully hidden.

We remind the reader that an x-ray is a two-dimensional image, but scoliosis is a three-dimensional deformity; furthermore, the modern transfer of reports to digital format makes measurement more difficult than traditional film methods and increases the margin of error, as the image is not true. For proper measurement, the accuracy of the metric scale of the image is fundamental (graphical representations on scales smaller than life increase the possibility of margins of error in interpretation).

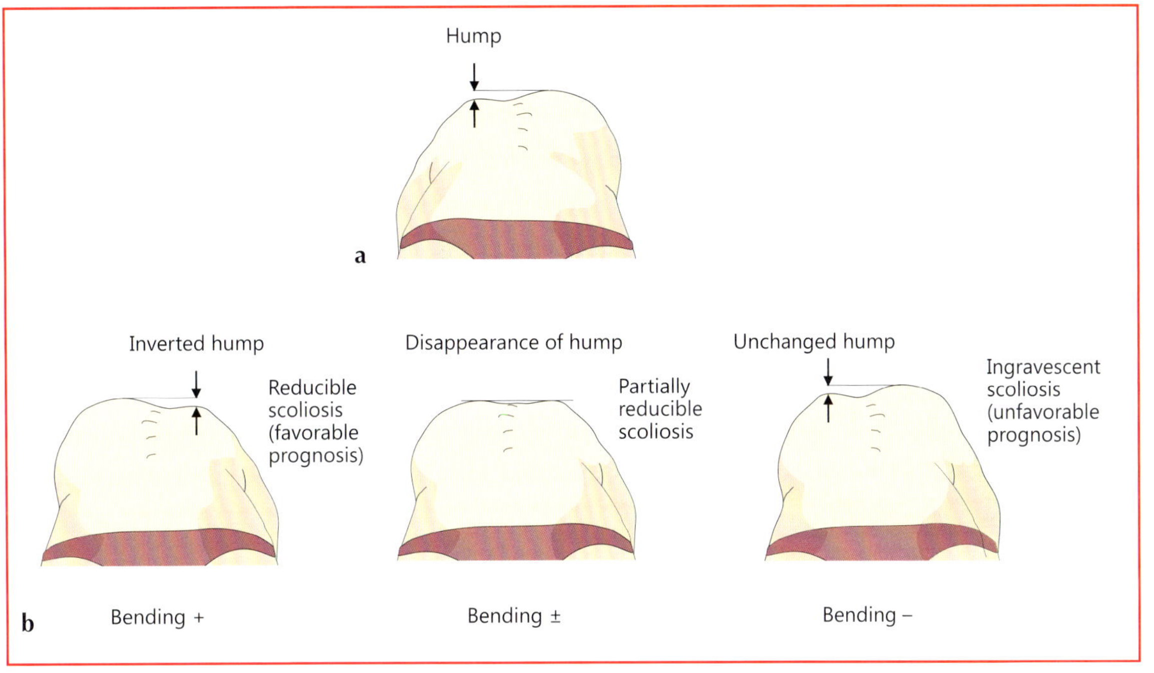

Figure 2.14 - Evaluation of the reducibility of the scoliotic curve going from the anterior bending position (**a**) to lateral bending (**b**) in the three cases of complete reducibility, incomplete reducibility, and non-reducibility.

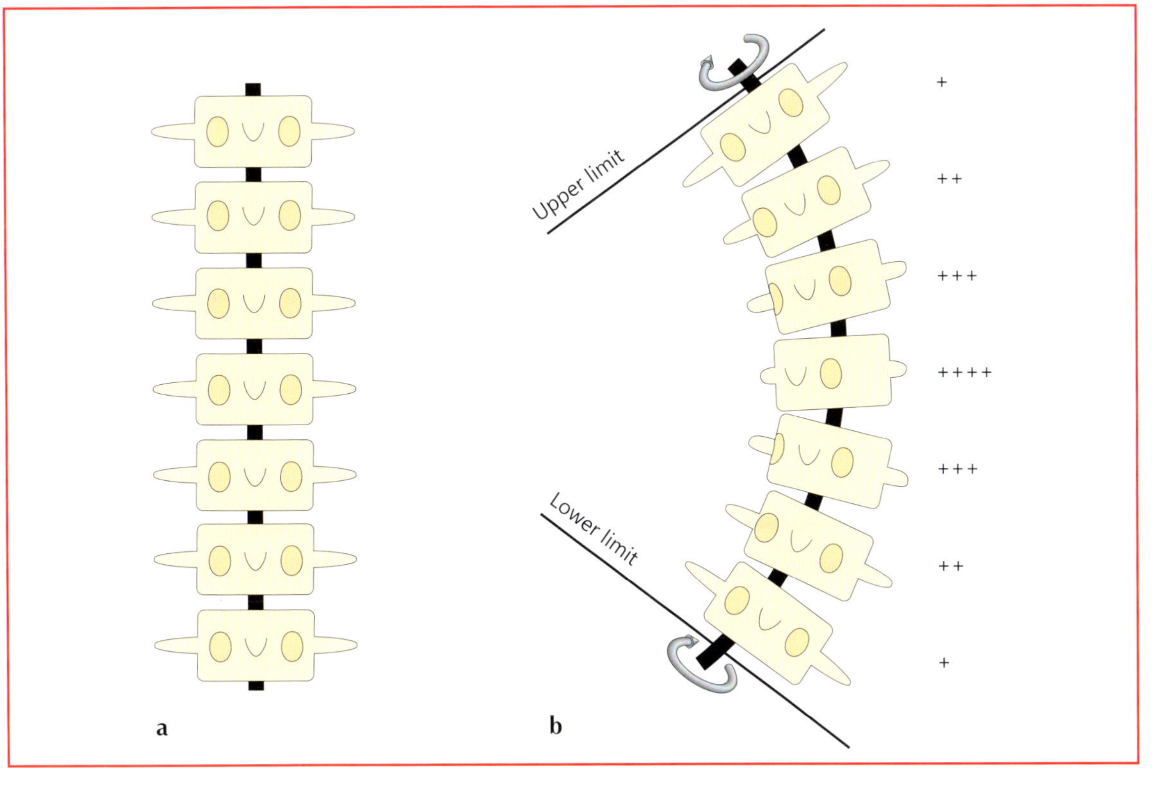

Figure 2.15 - Degree of rotation of the vertebral peduncles: frontal diagram view of physiological spinal column (**a**) and with structural scoliosis (**b**).

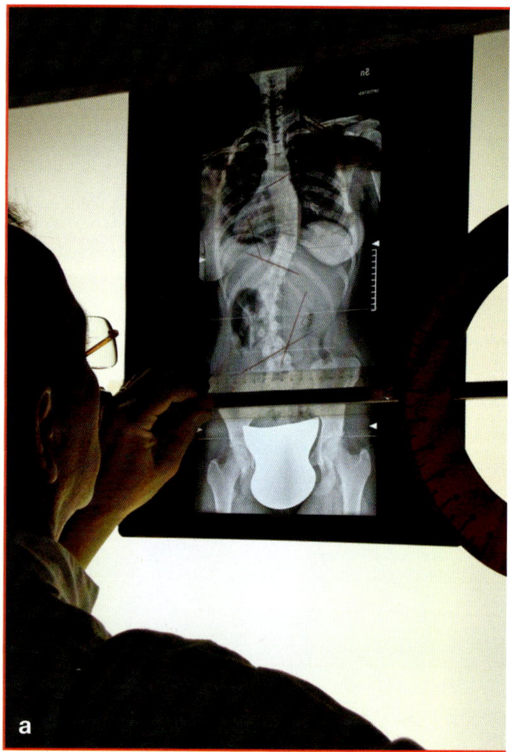

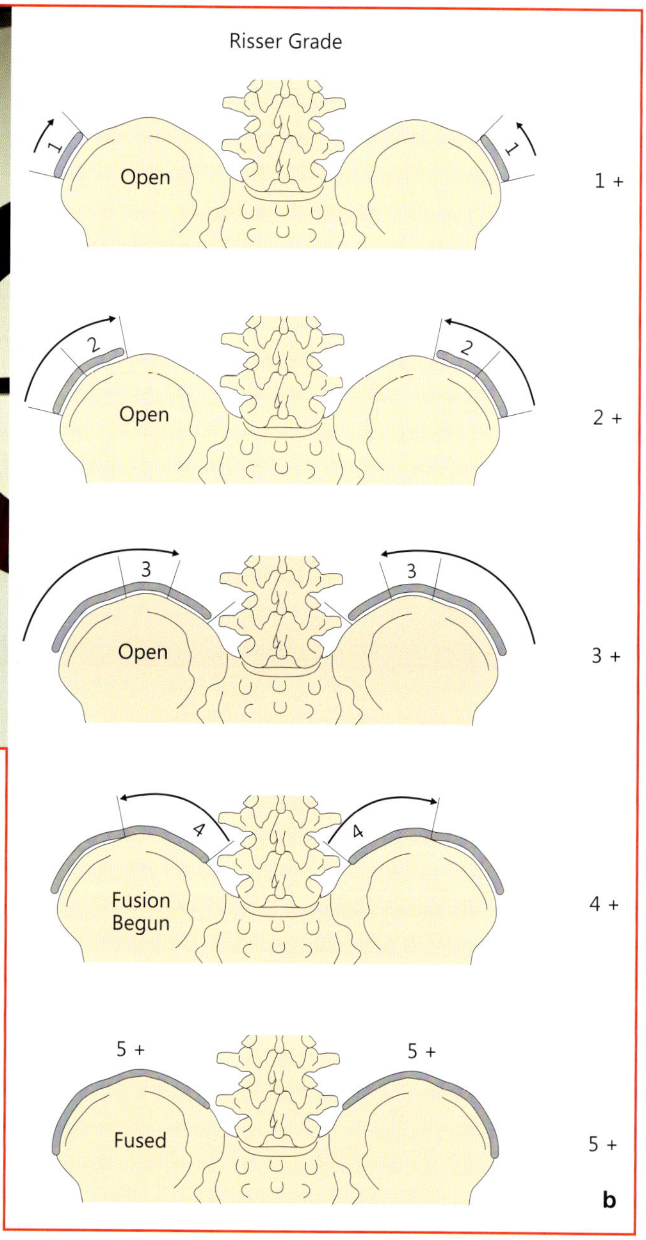

Figure 2.16 - From the x-ray, the state of maturity of the skeleton is determined (**a**) based on the Risser test (**b**).

Today there exist reports that analyze the spine in three dimensions, such as raster stereography, which is an extremely precise and less invasive analysis.

2.2.10 Risser Test

In order to determine the index of bone maturity, an x-ray of the pelvis is used to observe the presence or lack of the nucleus of ossification of the iliac crest, as it progresses up to fusion with the wing of ilium (figure 2.16). The term "Risser sign" indicates the various states of ossification: from the absence of the nucleus to its appearance (Risser 1), the formation of more nuclei (Risser 2), their fusion laterally to the crest (Risser 3), the medial extension (Risser 4), up to fusion with the ilium (Risser 5, full bone maturity).

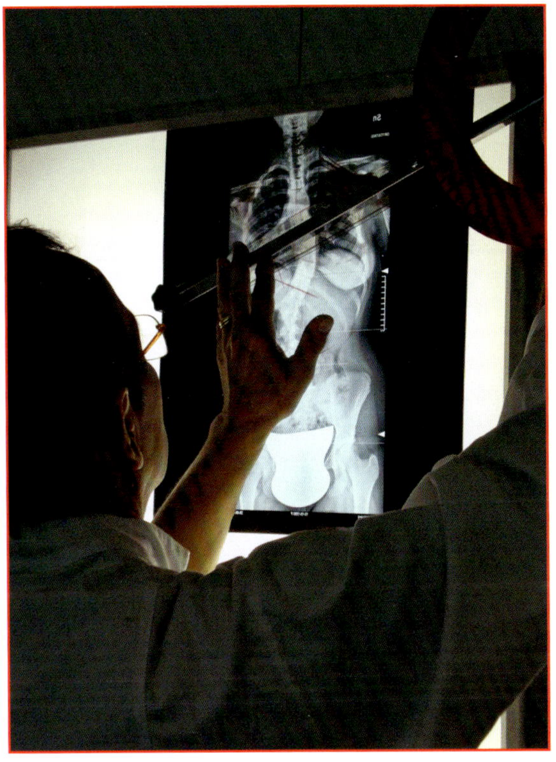

Figure 2.17 - Observation of the obliqueness of the ribs performed on the x-ray image, showing the longitudinal axis of the ribs themselves.

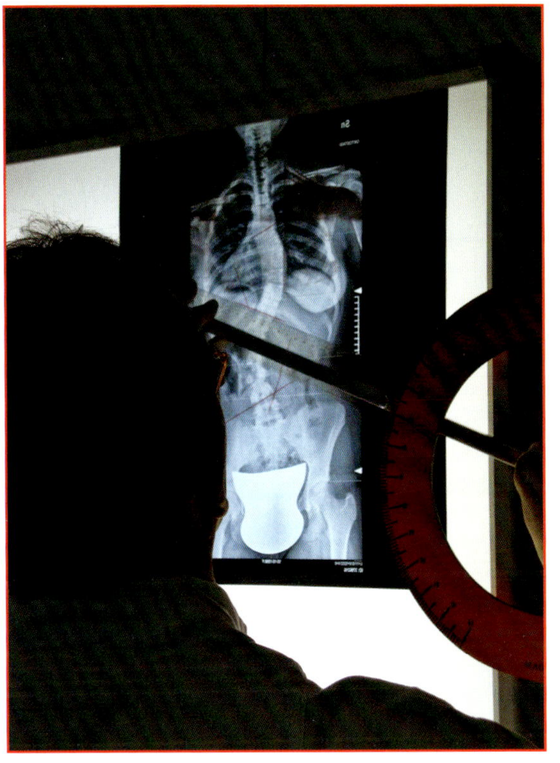

Figure 2.18 - Measurement of Cobb angle: find the upper and lower terminal vertebrae and trace the lines perpendicular to their transverse axes; these intersect to form the angle of the curve.

2.2.11 Observation of Obliqueness of Ribs

This observation is also done on the x-ray image, in frontal view. The examination verifies the extent of horizontalization of the ribs on the concave side, and verticalization of the ribs on the convex side of the scoliotic curve (figure 2.17).

2.2.12 Measurement of Scoliosis, Cobb Angle

Measurement with the Magri Cobbmeter is made on the frontal teleradiography, reducing the possibility of human error. The device significantly facilitates proper measurement. With the instrument, the two straight lines delimiting the upper and lower terminal vertebrae are sought. The sum of the two measurements gives the degree of scoliotic curvature (figure 2.18). The measurement may also be obtained with the goniometer, after having found the straight lines perpendicular to the two delimiting lines. The intersection of the two lines indicates the degree of scoliotic curvature.

2.2.13 Measurement of Lordotic Curvature Angle

This measurement, made on a teleradiography in laterolateral view, is obtained by aligning the Magri Cobbmeter instrument with the upper delimiting vertebra of the kyphotic convexity and then with the lower delimiting vertebra. An analogous measurement is made for the lordotic curve. Once the straight lines tangential to the upper and lower delimiting lines are traced, the Magri Cobbmeter allows for the quick and direct reading of the kypholordotic curve's value in degrees (figure 2.19).

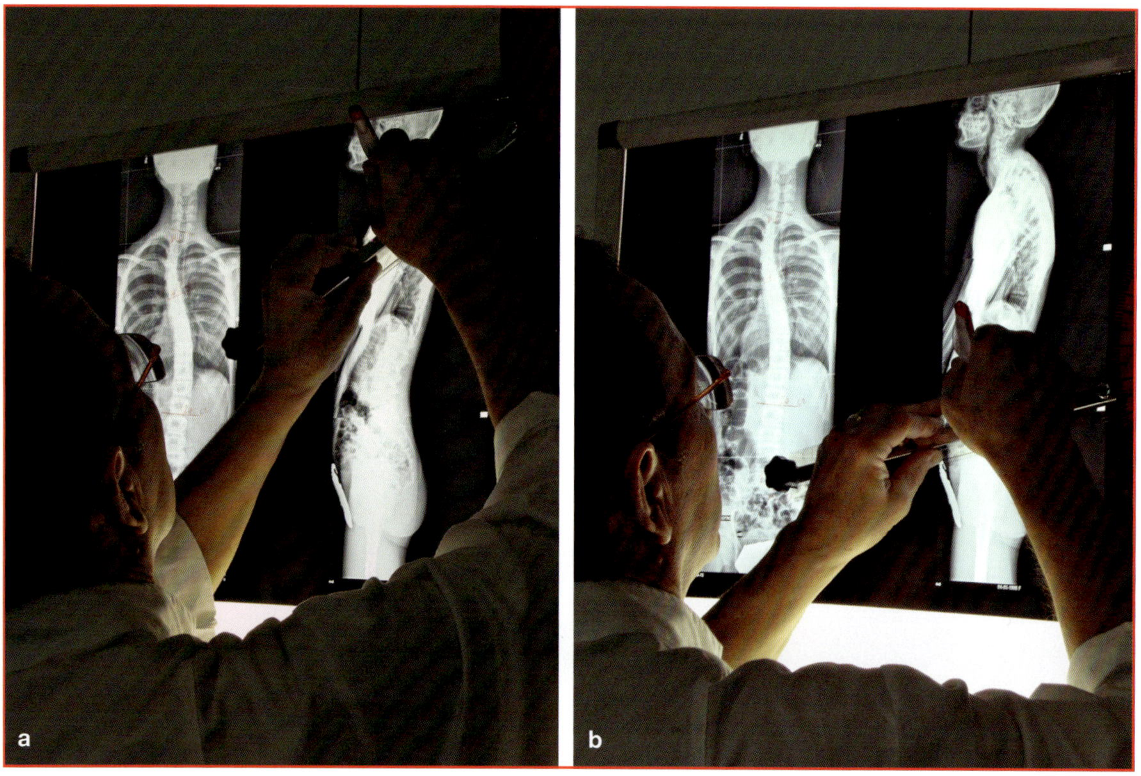

Figure 2.19 - Measurement of the angle of kypholordotic curvature: kyphotic curve (**a**); lordotic curve (**b**).

2.3 FUNCTIONAL KINESIOLOGICAL EXAMINATION

The functional kinesiological examination evaluates the patient's joint mobility and muscular tone-trophism. The aim of the examination is not an assessment that may be assimilated into the medical-orthopedic or clinical examination, but gives the kinesiologist the ability to implement and continually update personalized work in the gym. The examination suggested by the Rovatti Method® is enacted via a series of evaluations, described below. The figures show, if necessary, the same test performed on two patients, with two cases of scoliosis of different severity. The immediacy of the comparison allows for easier comprehension of the presented assessments.

2.3.1 Hypoextensibility of the Psoas

The examination is performed in the supine position, with the sacrum placed at the edge of the table. The limb to be examined (the right limb in figure 2.20) is allowed to fall passively in order to evaluate its tension. The left limb is pulled toward the chest in order to avoid any lumbar compensation that would make the test invalid.

2.3.2 Retroversion of the Pelvis and Abdominal Hold

In the supine position on the table, the patient keeps the knees flexed. Before performing the test, the patient must be taught how to approach and maintain the position of the pelvis in retroversion: contraction of the perineal muscle and simultaneous retroversion of the pelvis.

Once the proper retroversion position is reached, small lifts of the head and arms are assumed and held, until strong tension is felt in the abdominal muscles (primarily the rectus abdominis muscles). The examination assesses the abdominal hold, the kyphotization of the vertebral column, and muscle tone (figure 2.21).

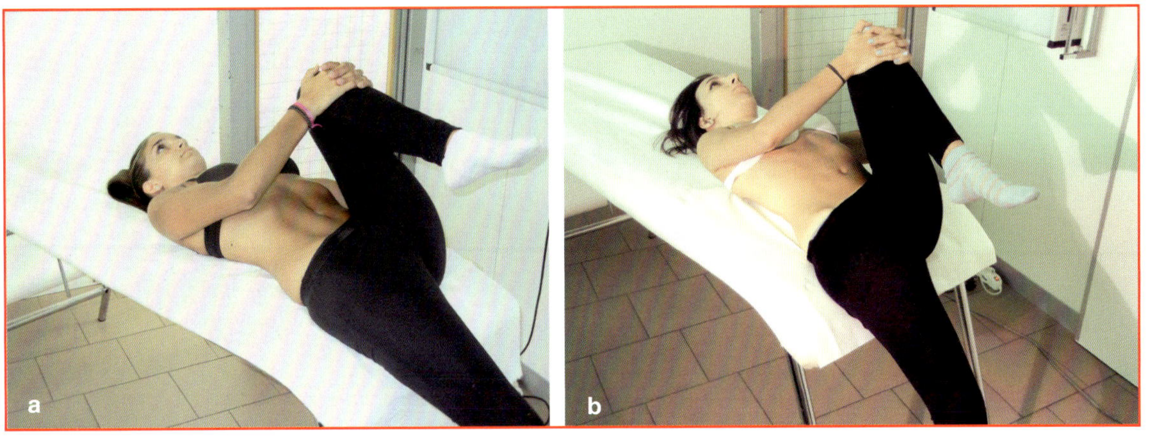

Figure 2.20 - Functional kinesiological examination: hypoextensibility of the psoas muscle. More toned muscle (**a**) renders the extension of the psoas more difficult. Looser muscle (**b**) facilitates the patient's ability to perform extreme extension.

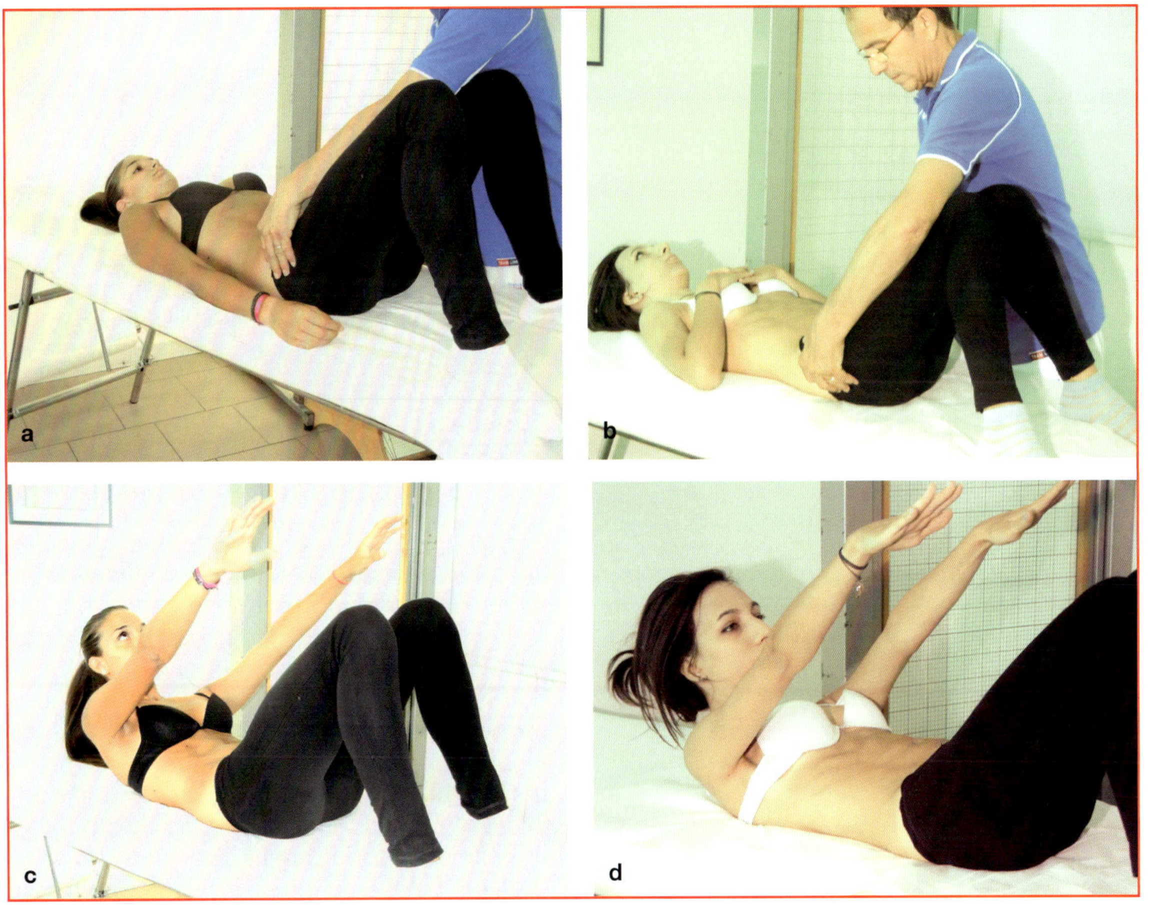

Figure 2.21 - Functional kinesiological examination: learning of the pelvic retroversion position in the two previously illustrated cases (**a**, **b**); evaluation of abdominal hold. The patient (**c**) succeeds in reaching kyphosis, while in the second case (**d**), with a more severe diagnosis of scoliosis, the patient shows difficulty in bringing the spine into kyphosis (case of structured flat dorsum).

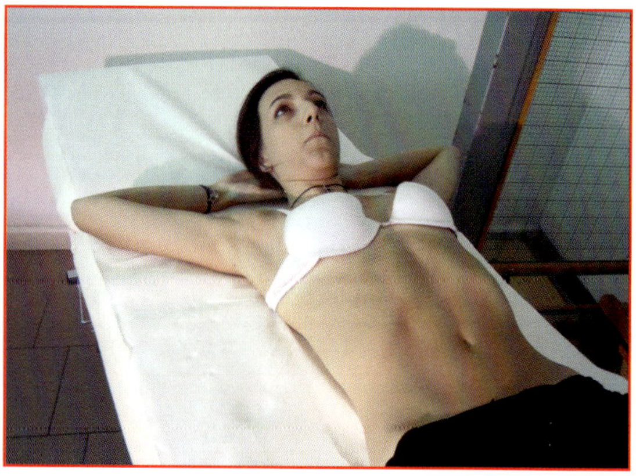

Figure 2.22 - Functional kinesiological examination: retraction of the pectoral muscles.

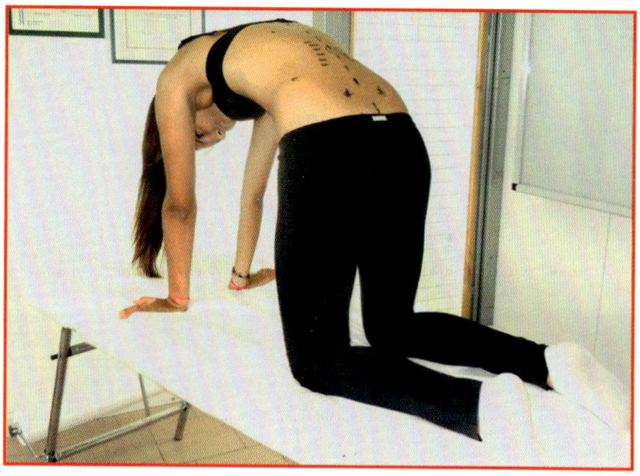

Figure 2.23 - Functional kinesiological examination: active kyphotization.

2.3.3 Anterior Bending of the Trunk

The test of anterior bending of the trunk, also known as the bending test or Adam's test, is performed not only for the measurement of humps and the evaluation of the reducibility of the curve, but also for the functional assessment of the spine and of the dorsal spine's capability for kyphotization.

2.3.4 Retraction of Pectoral Muscles (Pelvis in Retroversion)

The examination assesses the hypoextensibility of the pectoral muscles. It is performed on the table, with the patient in the supine decubitus position with the knees flexed (figure 2.22).

2.3.5 Active Kyphotization

The active kyphotization of the dorsal spine is particularly important. The patient is on the table in quadruped position. The weight is distributed evenly onto the arms and legs, with the hands extrarotated in order to facilitate the shoulders' participation in the exercise. The patient is asked to actively induce kyphosis (the back is rounded), with the pelvis kept in retroversion (figure 2.23).

2.3.6 Lateral Active Inclination

The test is carried out with the patient standing upright, and is assessed on the posterior frontal plane. The body is inclined laterally, alternately to the right and the left, and the distance from hand to ground is measured with the measuring stick in order to evaluate the flexibility of the trunk on the frontal plane and any asymmetries between the left and right sides (figure 2.24).

2.3.7 Ocular-motor Test

The patient is asked to perform several small jumps from one foot to the other, simultaneously exchanging a baton between one hand and the other. This test evaluates the capability for hand-eye control and coordination (figure 2.25).

2.3.8 Coordinative Ability Evaluation Test

Finally, several tests are performed for evaluating the patient's coordinative ability (coordination, rhythm, dexterity, balance) and any lacking aspects of the proprioceptive system or deficiencies in sensory, proprioceptive, or labyrinth-based information, as many subjects have balance problems. There are several examples of the tests performed: in the prone horizontal position, balancing on one stiff leg (alternately right and left), assess the ability to hold balance for at least 10 seconds; standing upright, balancing on a single leg with the other lifted, the patient is asked to keep balance for approximately ten seconds. In this case as well, the test is repeated by lifting one limb and then the other (figure 2.26).

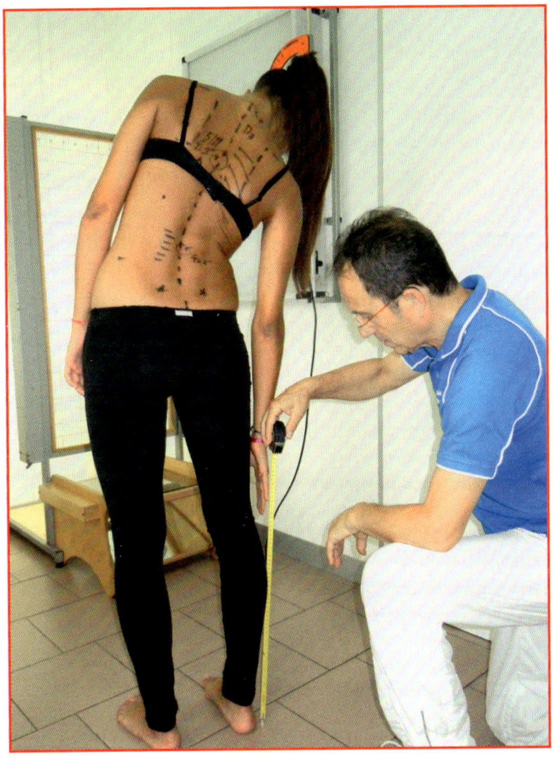

Figure 2.24 - Functional kinesiological examination: measurement of the lateral bending of the upper torso (trunk mobility) on the frontal plane.

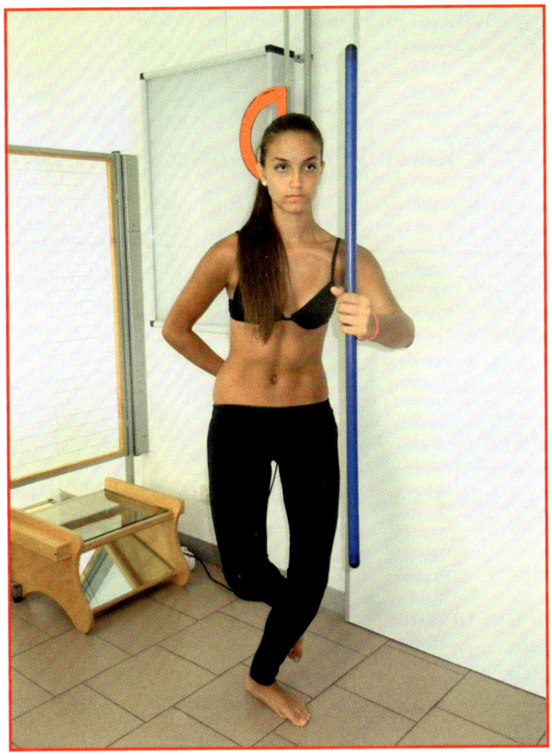

Figure 2.25 - Functional kinesiological examination: ocular-motor test.

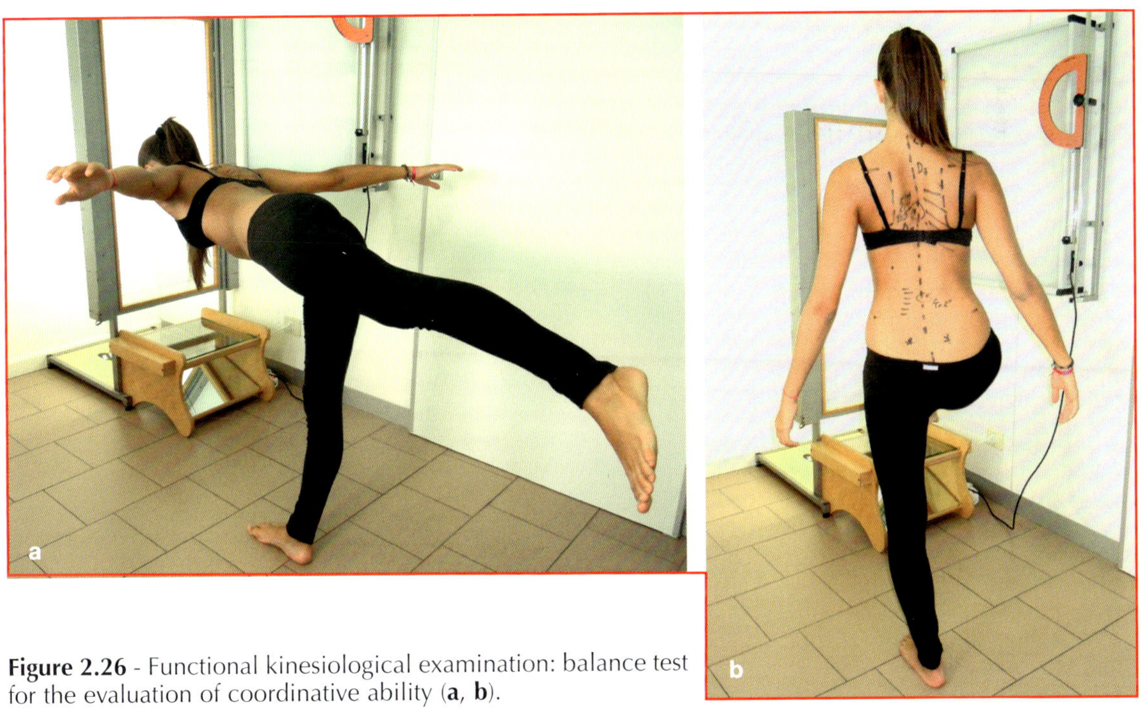

Figure 2.26 - Functional kinesiological examination: balance test for the evaluation of coordinative ability (**a**, **b**).

The tests are performed with the eyes open, and then are repeated with the eyes closed.

2.4 EVALUATION OF POSSIBLE ORTHOPEDIC CORSET

If the specialist has prescribed an orthopedic corset, the therapist or the kinesiologist must create a report sheet at the end of the evaluation session including indications of usage, dietary instructions, analisys and the comparison of orthopedic-physiatric data.

2.5 COUNSELING

In cases of kinesiotherapeutic treatment for the correction of idiopathic scoliosis that involve juveniles and adolescents, a counseling service should be implemented for the purposes of active involvement of the other family members, beginning from an initial informative meeting with the adolescents and their family. The assuming of responsibility by the family members for the management and treatment of the adolescent patient's scoliosis is fundamental. The family should be provided with pertinent responses in regards to the corrective plan, the duration of vertebral kinesiological treatment, the specific and personalized work plan being implemented, and the objectives of the work itself.

It is to be reiterated, in fact, that adolescent patients with scoliosis may have psychological problems due not only to deformity or scoliosis itself, but also to the difficulty in accepting the therapeutic and rehabilitative path proposed (in particular the orthopedic prescription of the corset). In our experience, work in professional teams has given the best results. The team should be comprised of all professional figures who may be necessary for the patient: in addition to the kinesiologist and the orthopedic specialist, the orthopedic technician, the physiotherapist, the gnathologist, and the psychologist.

Table 2.1 Objectives of Personalized Work

• Greater understanding of one's own body
• Study of one's own body in space
• Strengthening of the abdominal musculature, particularly the transverse and oblique muscles
• Improvement of the coordinative ability for developing greater exteroceptive and proprioceptive sensitivity (joint, tendinous and muscular receptors)
• Awareness of defects
• Greater muscular strengthening in the trunk for greater vertebral stability
• Search for greater postural tone to reduce any failure under loads
• Focused attention on work during exhalation for a better shaping effect
• Execution of work as much diversified as possible, seeking a good aesthetic aspect in order to attain greater psychological motivation and therefore more active participation in one's own specific work program

2.6 PERSONALIZED WORK PLAN AND KINESIOLOGICAL PROTOCOL

For proper implementation of the corrective protocol once the types of exercises to be performed and their possible sequence have been chosen (which must necessarily be personalized), the therapist, based on his or her own technical knowledge and experience, adapts the parameters relative to the intensity, duration, rhythm, and difficulty of each exercise, carrying out periodic check-ups (table 2.1). The exercises shall constantly be evaluated and possibly modified by the therapist, who will take care to introduce new ones as the patient's capabilities for proprioception increase and the patient acquires new abilities. Several corrective exercises that require the use of two or more elastic bands simultaneously in fact require a certain degree of proprioceptive experience and consciousness of the exercises on the patient's part.

The data found in the postural-functional kinesiological examination are necessary to assess several parameters of greater interest for the implementation of the working protocol. The exercises chosen are oriented toward overall-type kinesiotherapy.

3

Rovatti Method®

Acquiring consciousness of one's own posture, reactions, and compensations in order to then correct, refine, and internalize a new, correct body scheme: this is, in brief summary, the approach and objective of the specific work programs of the Rovatti Method®.

The theoretical basis of the Rovatti Method® is derived from the Lyon school, and begins from these base concepts in order to propose new methods and to reach the indicated goals.

The use of elastic bands is studied and applied as a possibility for rehabilitating and reshaping the spine, seeking correction on all three planes of space. The elastic bands are used as if they were the therapist's hands: they envelop and shape the area to be treated, teaching the patient to perceive, internalize, and self-correct.

3.1 SEARCH FOR NEW BODY SCHEME

Posture is the final result of a **complex motor coordination process** that involves the synergistic action of the various physiological, neurosensory, and muscular systems, as Sibilla always used to reiterate. In dynamic conditions, good posture and kinetic coordination are a prerequisite for a "perfected" voluntary motor act i.e., exactly what constitutes the objective of a medical exercise.

In the case of vertebral pathologies, dysmorphism and true scoliosis, a corrective therapeutic path must be defined with the objective of constructing a body scheme and thus proper posture. The therapist (with the support of the entire therapeutic team) and the patient work together to reach this end, implementing an **individual and personalized program** based on the person's requirements, age, and pathological condition.

The central core of the work, which may also be performed in a gym in small groups, is made up of exercises performed with the use of elastic bands (the bases are illustrated below). In addition to this, the personalized work requires general and specific motor activity and exercises for the development of aerobic capacity performed without the use of the elastic bands. An additional supplementary part of the rehabilitative protocol proposed comprises ergonomic data and proper performance of motor act so that these may be repeated in daily life and become proper habits beyond the gym and the specific treatment times.

Ergonomics, by definition, is a technique that analyzes, assesses, and structures simple or complex systems that require interaction with a human operator, using knowledge of a biomedical, engineering, and psychosocial nature. In the field of medical exercise, ergonomics is synonymous (both static and dynamic) with musculoskeletal function in full respect of the physiology of osteoarticular structures and in the performance of motor act. The integration between the support structures of the vertebral column, of a passive (vertebrae, discs, ligaments) and active nature (neuromuscular apparatus), is translated into movement. With physiological spinal curvature, biomechanical functionality causes a reduction in muscular effort, using the force of gravity in order to control and modulate muscle contraction.

Additionally, relaxation techniques aimed at

reducing psycho-muscular tension (which often accompanies the clinical situation of scoliosis patients) are useful to complete the program. In the gym, easy relaxation techniques can be performed, guided by the therapist's voice, in ideal ergonomic conditions. The patient maximum attention is required, and they are invited to take consciousness of their own body, their contact with the floor, and their natural respiration, putting them "at ease". The aim is to have tension reduced and attenuated. Often, vertebral pains that influence proper posture are caused by anxiety, stress, and poor management of one's own body.

3.2 TREATMENT WITH THE USE OF ELASTIC BANDS

The peculiarity and the positive aspect of the Rovatti Method® reside in the use of elastic bands as if they were the therapist's hands, shaping the spine in three dimensions. The perception of the forces provided by the elastic allows for greater sensitization to correction. During the performance of exercises, **respiration occurs in two phases**: an initial, brief inhalation phase in preparation for exercise, and a second, slow and prolonged exhalation phase to allow for the reduction of tension in the contraction of the thoracic muscles due to the elasticity of the osteoarticular structures and the pulmonary parenchyma.

Table 3.1 Elastic Bands: Purpose of Use

• Refine balance reactions
• Facilitate the awareness
• Improve postural correction
• Develop a motor pattern in respiratory exercises
• Facilitate better shaping
• Have better precision in corrective asymmetrical exercises and strengthening symmetrical exercises
• Correct the spinal column with non-compensated stretching exercises
• Facilitate greater understanding of corrective exercises in daily life

The selection of the elastic bands, which differ in resistance and color, is made by the therapist, who follows the patient in the preparation of corrective exercises. The same exercise done by persons of differing age, sex, height, strength and preparation will entail the use of different elastic bands, with the same efficacy. The choice of elastic bands used by the patients and models on the following pages should not be read as the only possibility for the exercises illustrated.

The destabilizing function and action of the elastic band is also a stimulus for neuromotor control, wherever there exist reductions of proprioceptive afference. Table 3.1 presents a summary of the goals that may be achieved through the use of elastic bands.

The elastic band is made of latex, hypoallergenic, highly extendable material. Its principal characteristics are convenience, safety, and adaptability in moving bony levers with progressive resistance. These properties allow auxotonic (increasing intensity), concentric, eccentric, and isometric actions to be performed with three-dimensional movements as well.

The elastic bands are made with materials of different intensity and resistance, recognizable by their range of colors (specific to each company that produces them): the therapist selects the density of the elastic band based on the type of subject to be treated and their morphological characteristics, as well as on the type of work that is to be performed.

3.2.1 Therapist-patient Relationship

For proper results of corrective exercises, the therapist's continuous observation of the exercise is a determining factor. The constant presence of the therapist for the visual improvement of the corrective exercise is indispensable. The progressive internalization of the proper motor act is required of the patient.

Therapist and patient actively collaborate to establish a new postural and motor scheme.

The work is individual and personalized, the experiences are shared.

Therapist and patient collaborate actively and continually for the establishment of the proper motor scheme, as well as for its repetition and internalization.

For this reason – the need of a continuous exchange and relationship between therapist and patient – the Rovatti Method® involves personalized work in a small-group context.

The preparation of the work arises from attentive static-dynamic evaluation of the person, or more precisely from the results of the postural and functional kinesiological examination, in addition to the information obtained by the therapeutic team.

The number of patients that may be incorporated into the group depends on both the therapist's capability and the patients' level of preparation.

3.2.2 Notes on Interpretation of Exercises

The exercises illustrated in the second part of this book (**Treatment with Elastic Bands: Specific Work Programs**) are the most important and widespread of those proposed to the patient, in our experience. It is helpful to remember that they are taken from personalized, specific protocols that were directed at one particular person. The exercises may thus be implemented into the personalized rehabilitative protocol of other patients, but, under the control of the therapist and the work team, adapted to specific cases.

The exercises, divided by type and severity of scoliosis, must thus be read as examples, in order to possibly establish other protocols.

Another substantial consideration: exercises with elastic bands, above all those of greater complexity (some involve the simultaneous use of three elastic bands), are aimed at **necessarily experienced patients**. That is, patients who have practiced corrective treatment for a long time and who have already developed a sufficient degree of understanding and bodily awareness, as well as that of proprioceptive stimulation and corrections, sometimes minimal, that have been required.

In the illustrations explaining the exercises, patients are shown with primary right dorsal and secondary left lumbar-dorsal scoliosis, as these are statistically the most widespread forms of scoliosis. Naturally, in the opposite situation (left dorsal and right dorsolumbar scoliosis), the therapist will have the exercise performed from the opposite side.
In the text, the male gender is always used, for reasons of simplicity.

Three-dimensional corrective exercises are performed during a slow and prolonged exhalation phase.

The other patients will progressively be introduced to the comprehension of the exercises, to an always-greater proprioceptive sensitivity of the reactions and corrections of their own body, until gaining complete consciousness and internalization of the proper motor act.

In order to clarify the principle of the method, figure 3.1 summarizes the three basic concepts: the three corrective movements to be performed in succession. Together, these establish the three-dimensional correction of the scoliotic curve sought with the exercises, and in particular with the help of the elastic bands: **kyphotization**, **lateralization,** and **derotation** of the dorsal spine, concepts that derive from the principles of Lyon exercise and the intuition of the three-dimensionality of scoliotic curves, from which arises correction on the three spatial planes.

The three corresponding forces that the patient seeks are shown by three-dimensional arrows in order to facilitate, where possible, their reading.

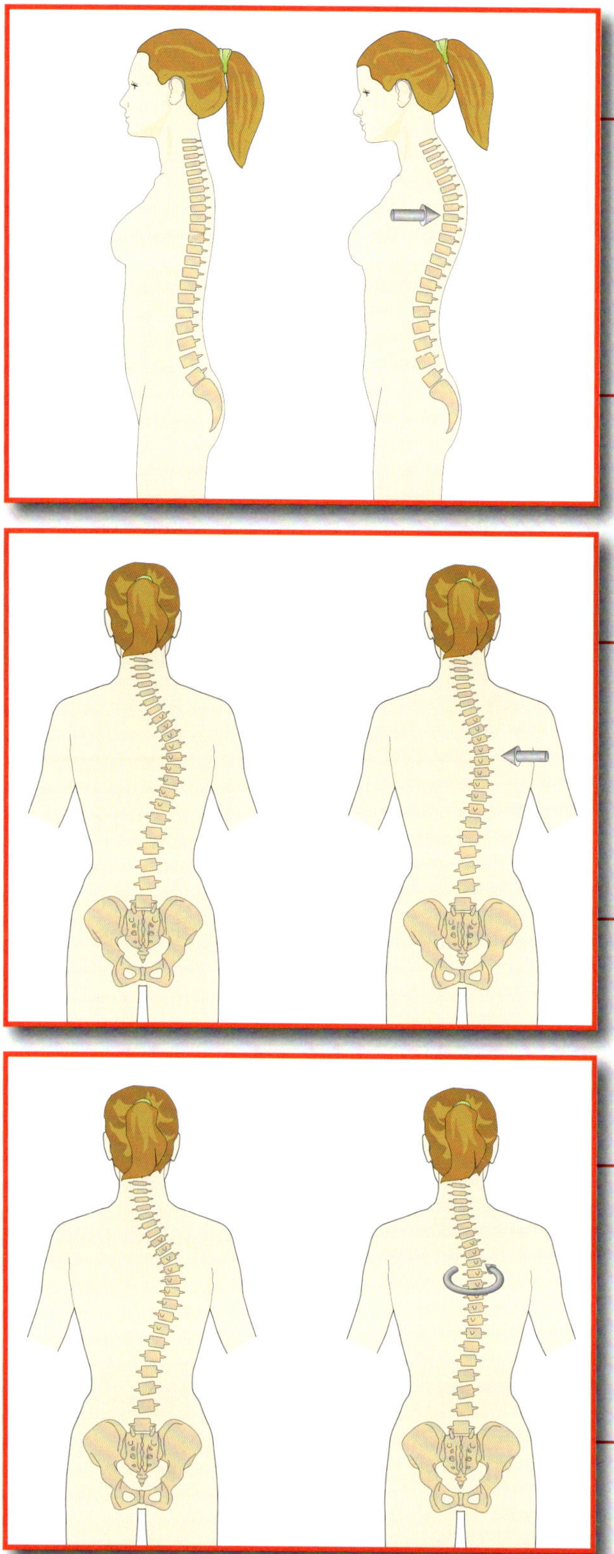

Kyphotization

The vertebral column is made convex on the sagittal plane (in search of physiological curve).

Lateralization

The spine moves laterally on the frontal plane from the side opposite to the hump.

Derotation

The vertebral column rotates on the longitudinal axis in an inverse manner to the rotation that causes the characteristic hump.

Figure 3.1 - Rovatti Method®: the three keywords. To the left is a schematic diagram of uncorrected scoliosis; to the right are the three moments of correction sought on the three spatial planes with the help of the elastic bands.

SECOND PART

Treatment with Elastic Bands: Specific Work Programs

4

Minor Scoliosis and Paramorphism

Work with elastic bands for the correction of minor scoliosis and paramorphism involves various exercise sequences aimed at gaining awareness of one's own posture, body's reactions and corrections, and improving body scheme.

Exercises may be included into the personalized rehabilitative protocol under the control of the therapist and the work team.

The exercises recommended for minor scoliosis and paramorphism are:

- balance reaction refinement exercises
- body scheme refinement exercises
- postural reactions and awareness
- anti-gravitational muscular strength and overall kinesiotherapy exercises
- strengthening symmetrical exercises
- correction exercises with the maintenance of posture and gaining awareness
- development exercises of a moderate aerobic capacity
- ergonomics exercises
- muscular stretching exercises
- general motor activity.

EXERCISE 4.1

Balance Reaction Refinement Exercises

These are destabilizing exercises aimed at the refinement of balance reactions and the development of proprioceptive sensitivity (perception of proprioceptive and exteroceptive stimuli).

Execution - On destabilizing podalic support with the use of a roller. The elastic band is placed under the roller; the patient pulls with the arms, seeking balance and good postural structure, verified by the patient with the use of mirrors both on the lateral plane (**a**) and on the frontal plane (**b**).

Variant - Destabilizing podalic support with the use of the roller as before; the elastic band is positioned under the feet, but not under the roller (**c**).

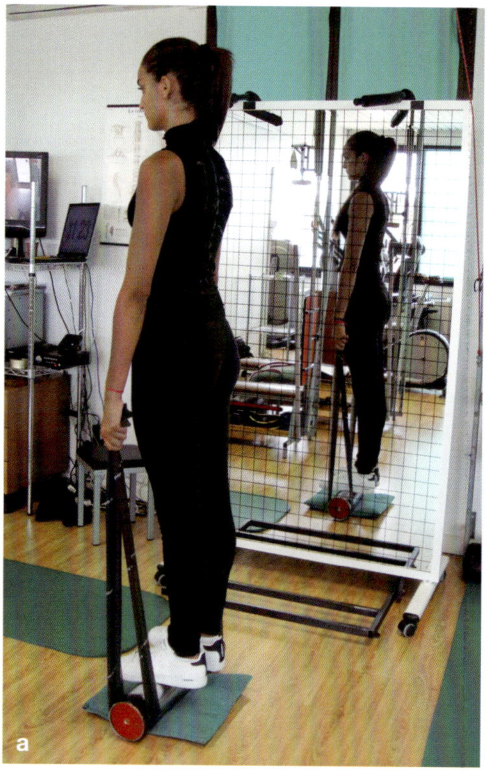

a

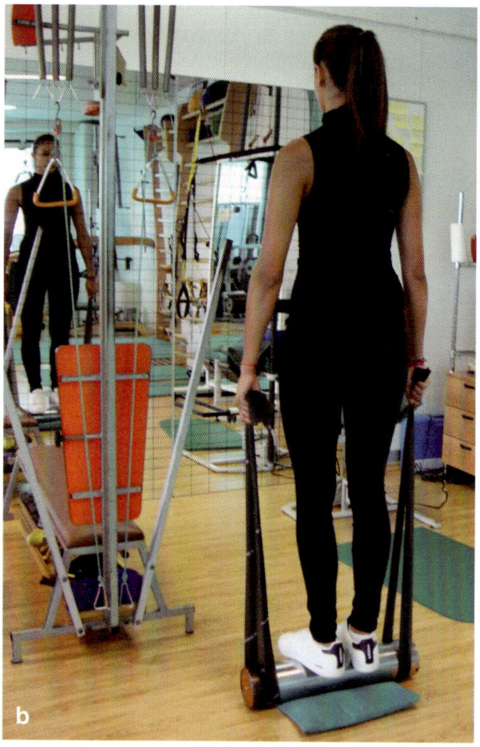

b

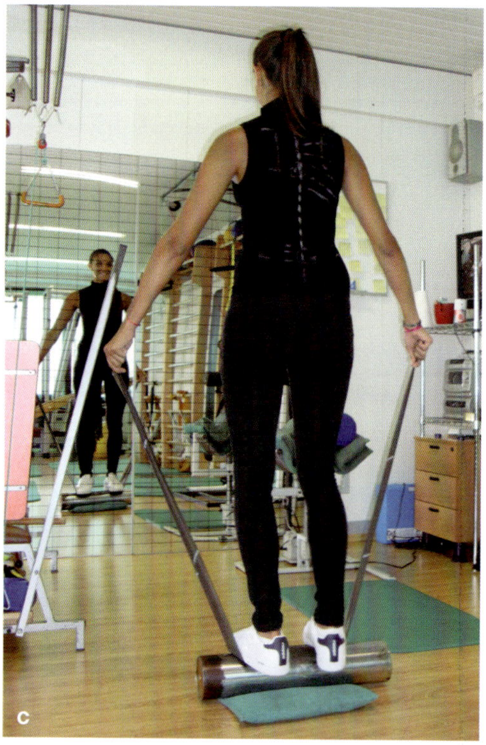

c

EXERCISE 4.2

Gaining Awareness of Defects

Self-analysis of posture and gaining awareness of defects. Laterolateral and anterior-posterior posture. Self-monitoring with the use of different mirrors is essential.

Execution - With the patient standing upright in front of the mirror, the elastic band is under the feet (which are held together) and kept with the hands, with the arms extended laterally. This exercise may be carried out with a baton on the head. The first phase is of control of the waist triangles; the second is the abduction of the upper limbs for corrective purposes.

a, Starting position; **b**, correction.

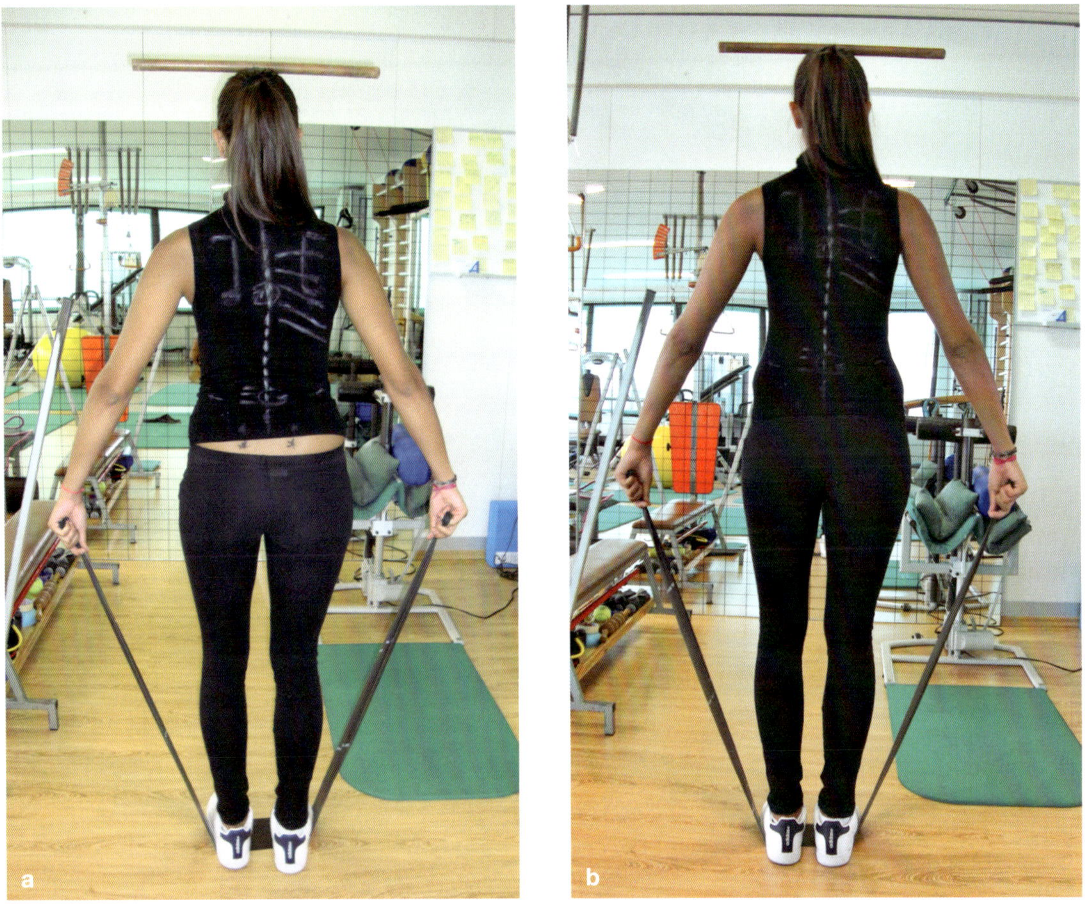

EXERCISE 4.3

Destabilization

The objective of this exercise is the refinement of the balance reaction and the development of proprioceptive sensitivity.

Execution - With the patient standing in a horizontal pronc position with only one foot on the ground to hold the elastic band, perform a lateral traction (**a**, **b**) while seeking balance and proper postural structure despite the unstable support. The exercise may also be performed while wearing the corset (**c**).

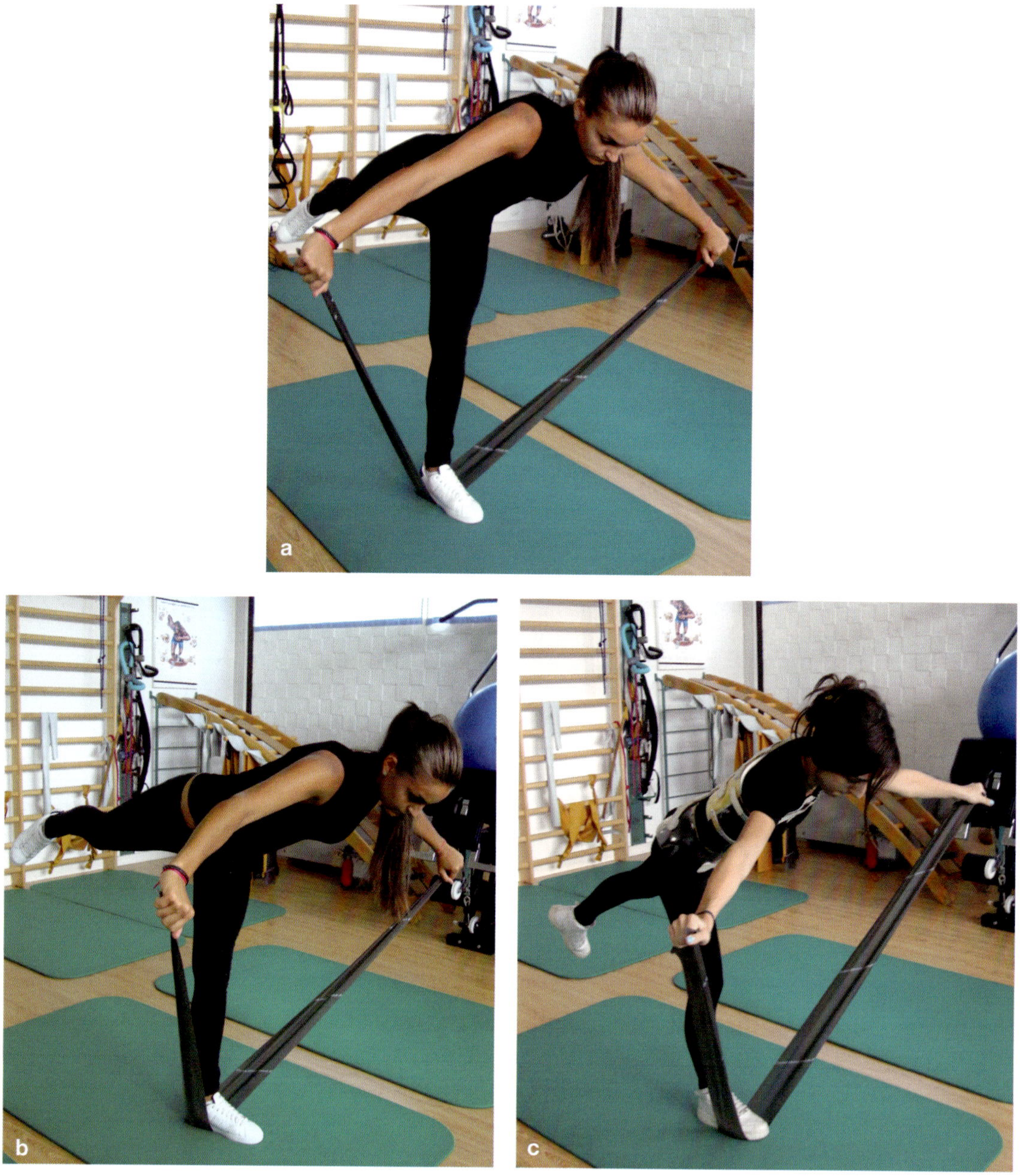

EXERCISE 4.4

Gaining Awareness of Defects

Self-analysis of posture and gaining awareness of defects. Laterolateral and anterior-posterior posture. Self-monitoring with the use of different mirrors is essential.

Execution - Sitting on the bench in front of the mirror with the elastic band under the gluteus and the arms extended laterally at the level of the shoulders. The left leg is lifted and resting on the bench.

a, Starting position;
b, kyphotization and lateralization;
c, derotation.

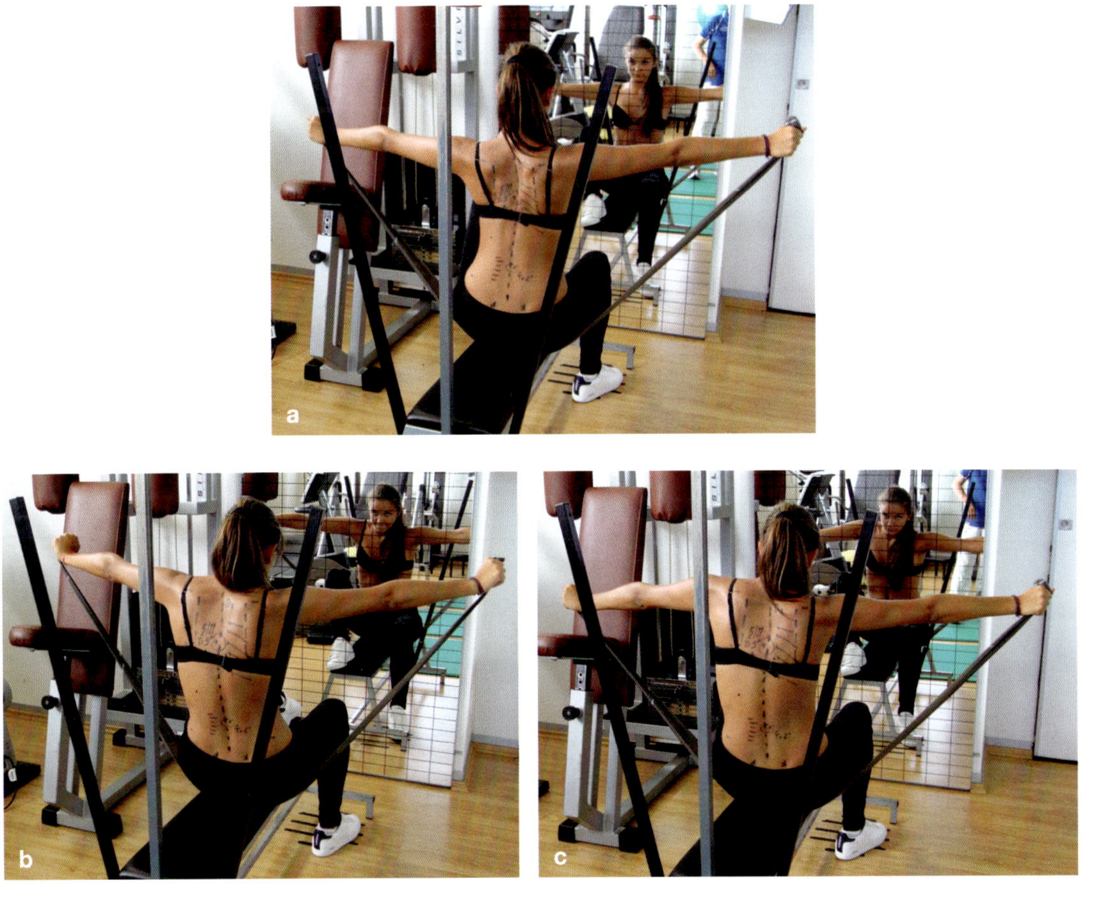

EXERCISE 4.5

Balance Reaction Refinement Exercises

This exercise acts on coordination, dexterity, rhythm, and balance.

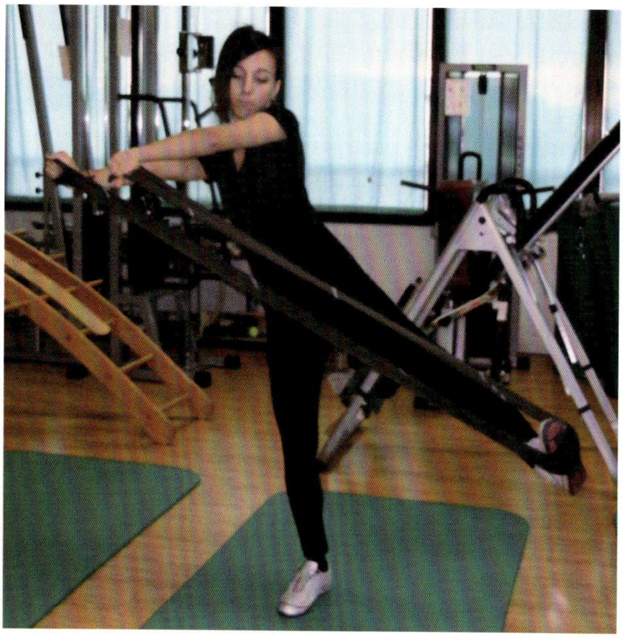

Execution - The elastic band is wrapped around the foot and the ends are held and pulled away from the foot by the hands. An opposed oscillation of the limbs that hold the elastic band is vigorously performed. The exercise is repeated with the other leg.

EXERCISE 4.6

Destabilization

An exercise that engages the patient in the development of coordinative capabilities.

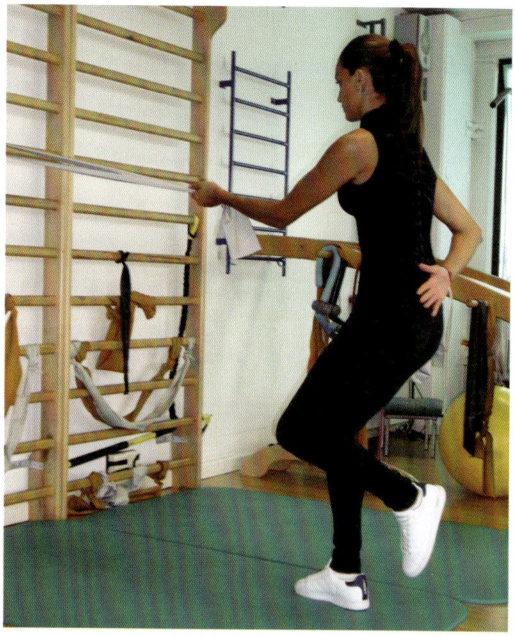

Execution - Traction of the elastic band fixed to the wall bars with coordinated changes of the hand and leg during small leaps. The elastic band is repeatedly passed between one hand and the other, and must remain constantly under traction.

EXERCISE 4.7

Mobilization

The objective of this exercise is the mobilization of the dorsolumbar spine.

Execution - On the knees with the elastic band beneath the knees, the patient slides alternately to the left and right, maintaining correct posture with the help of the elastic.

a, **b**, Anterior frontal view;
c, **d**, posterior view.

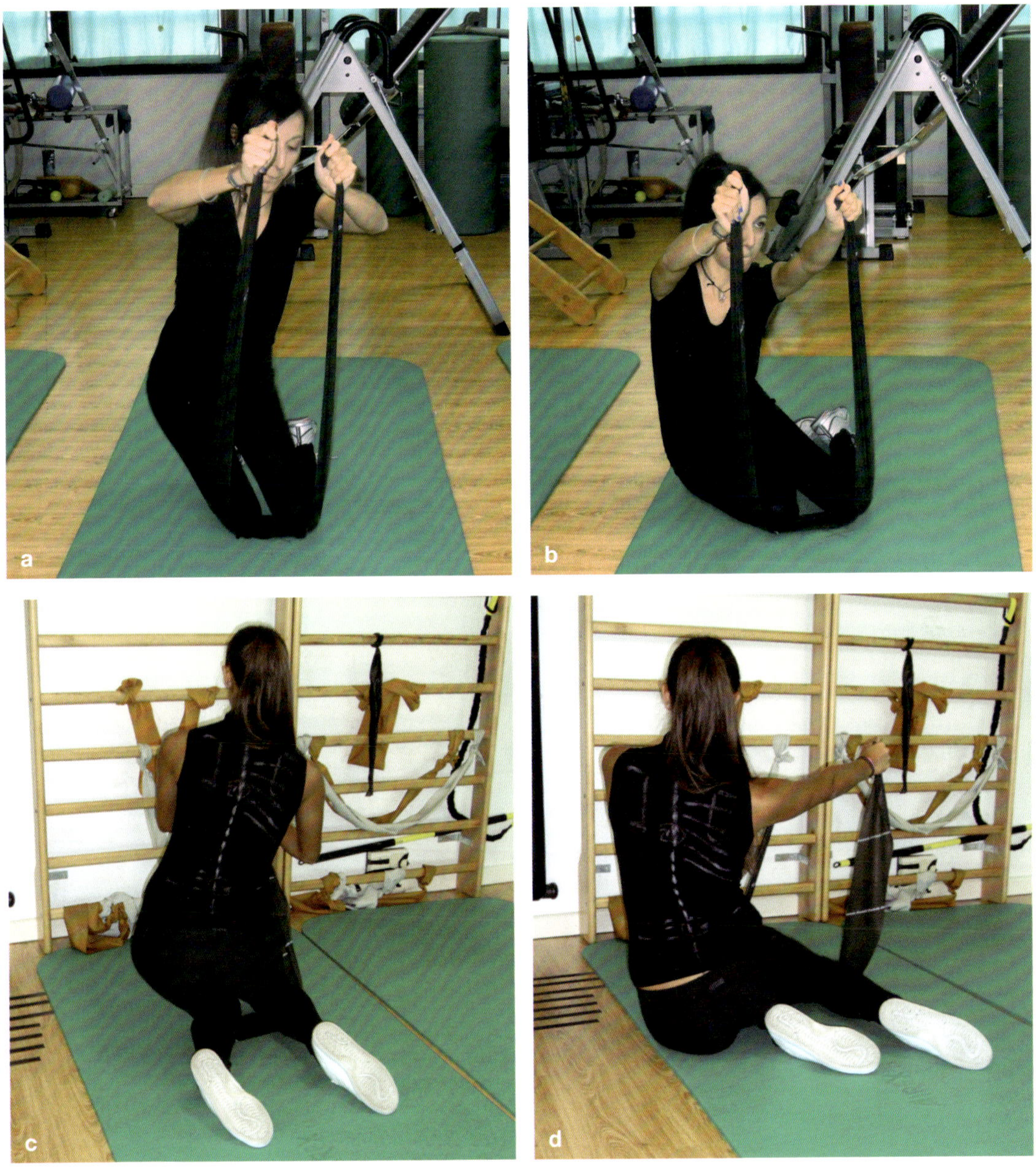

EXERCISE 4.8

Balance Reaction Refinement Exercises

The objective is the perception and refinement of proprioceptive stimuli.

Execution - With the patient lying supine on a roller, the elastic band is positioned under the back, wrapping it at the dorsal hump, and is held in tension by the hands at the two ends. The patient must maintain balance via spinal perception, sensing imbalances in the support and correcting them with the use of the elastic band.

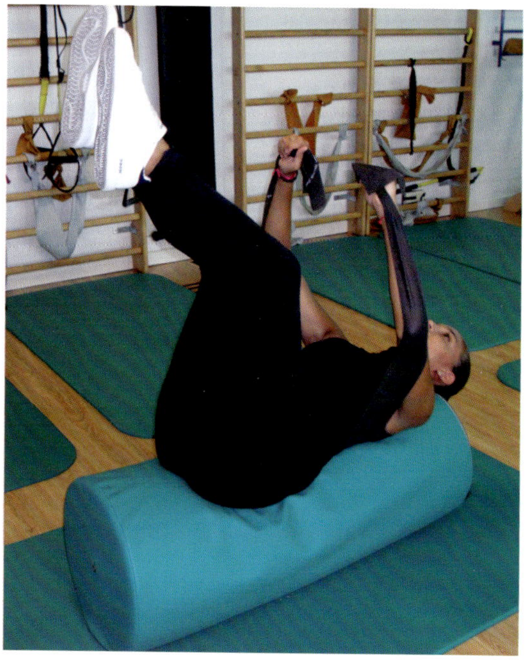

EXERCISE 4.9

Short Skip

The objective is the development of conditional abilities.

Execution - The skip is performed by keeping the elastic band fixed to the wall bars and positioned over the abdomen, under traction. The therapist may put a second elastic band in place to sum the elastic's forces of resistance.

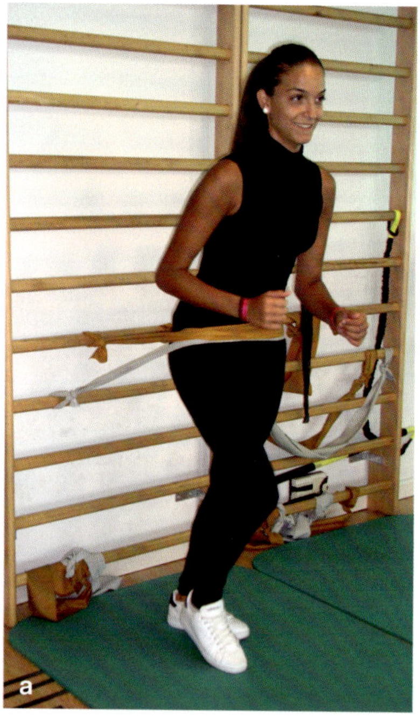

a

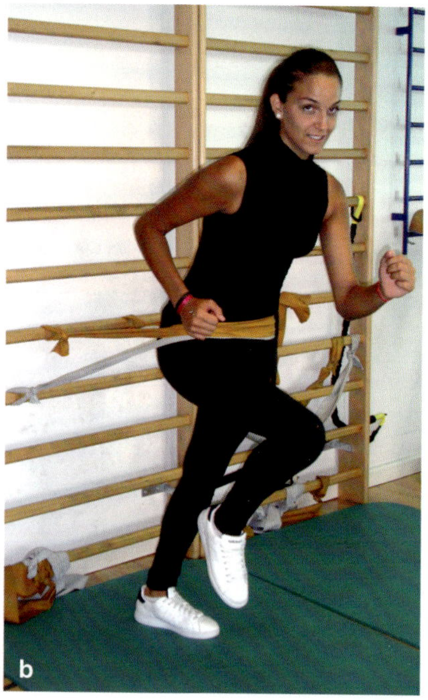

b

EXERCISE 4.10

Cross-country Skiing

This exercise develops the patient's cardio-respiratory capacity and achieve moderate muscular strengthening.

Execution - Rhythmic bending of the lower limbs, with alternating coordination of the upper limbs.

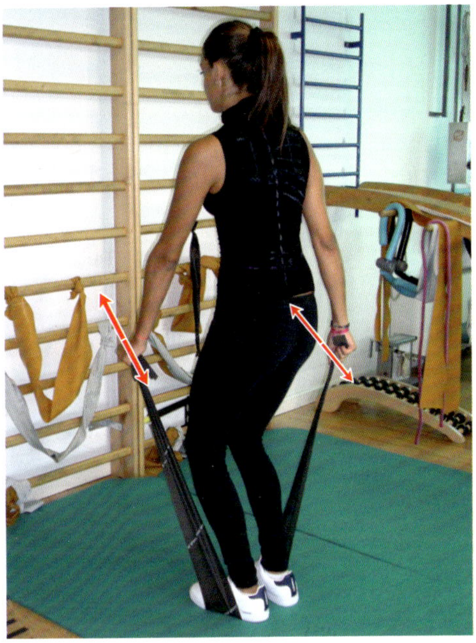

EXERCISE 4.11

Respiratory Exercise

Costal respiration against elastic resistance.

Execution - With the patient in the supine position with the legs lifted, the band is positioned under the back at the dorsal hump. Crossing the band in front of the chest and holding the ends with lateral extension of the upper limbs, the patient performs forced exhalation so as to reduce thoracic circumference (**a**). The patient then immediately induces tension with the elastic and lately inhales forcefully so as to obtain greater activation of the muscles used for this action (**b**).

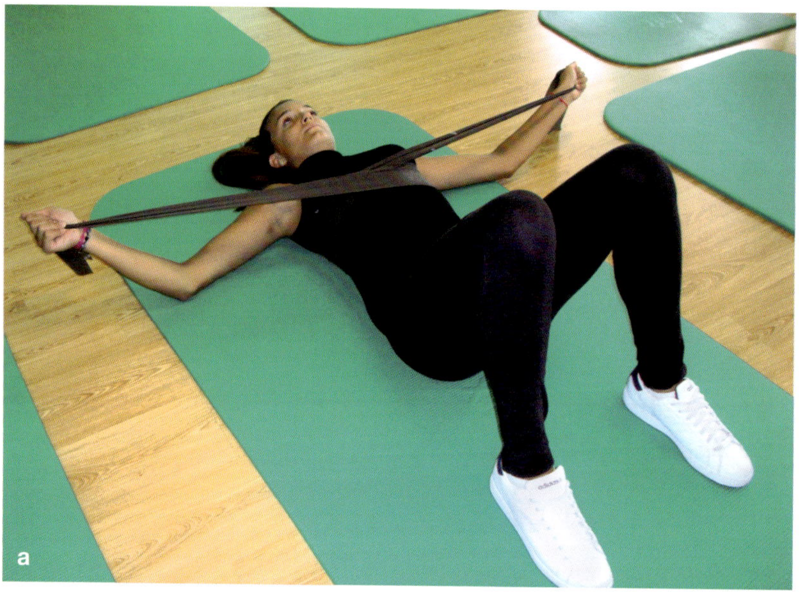

a

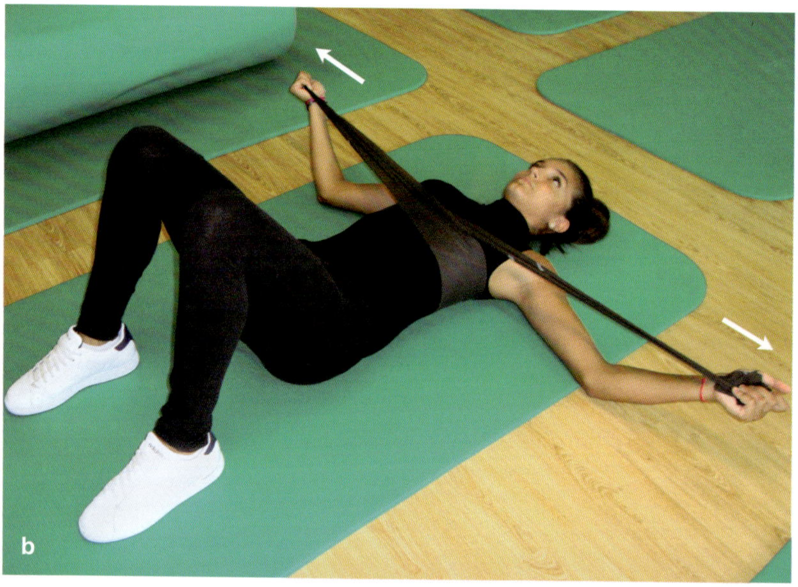

b

EXERCISE 4.12

Diaphragmatic Respiration

The objective of this exercise is expansion of the diaphragm against elastic resistance.

Execution - In the supine position with the legs lifted, as in the preceding exercise, the elastic band is positioned on the abdomen, having been passed under the back. The patient breathes, perceiving the progressive diaphragmatic expansion via the muscle activation in the state of opposing resistance.

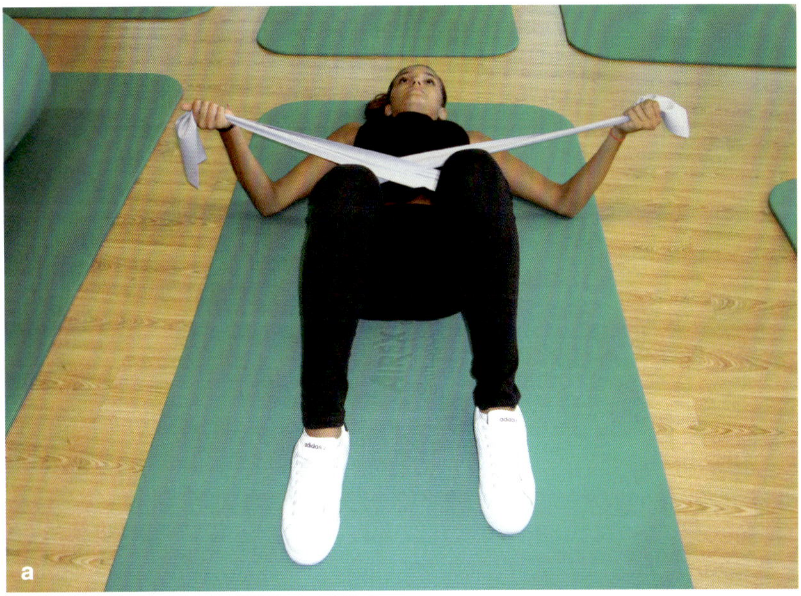
a

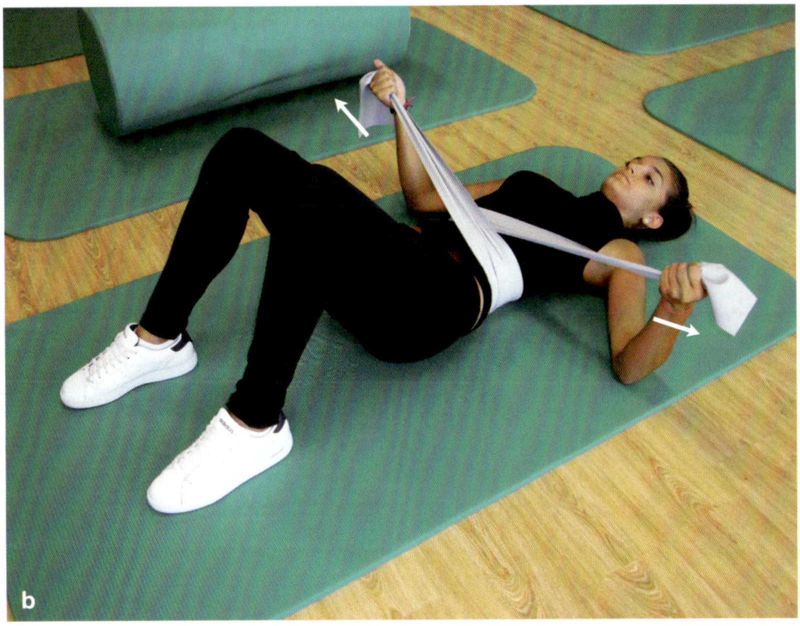
b

EXERCISE 4.13

Balance Reaction Refinement Exercises

The objective of this exercise is the control of balance reactions, the strengthening of the paravertebral muscles, and the activation of the correction of the right dorsal hump (via the three-dimensional correction of the spine).

Execution - On the knees, balancing on a Bobath ball (destabilizing element), the patient wraps the elastic band around the head and holds it between the hands, resting on the wall bars. The patient performs retropulsion of the head against elastic resistance in conditions of self-induced stretching of the spine.

Keeping the balance stable and the spine in a state of elongation, the patient seeks the three-dimensional correction of the spine through the three successive phases: kyphotization (**a**), lateralization (**b**), and finally derotation (**c**).

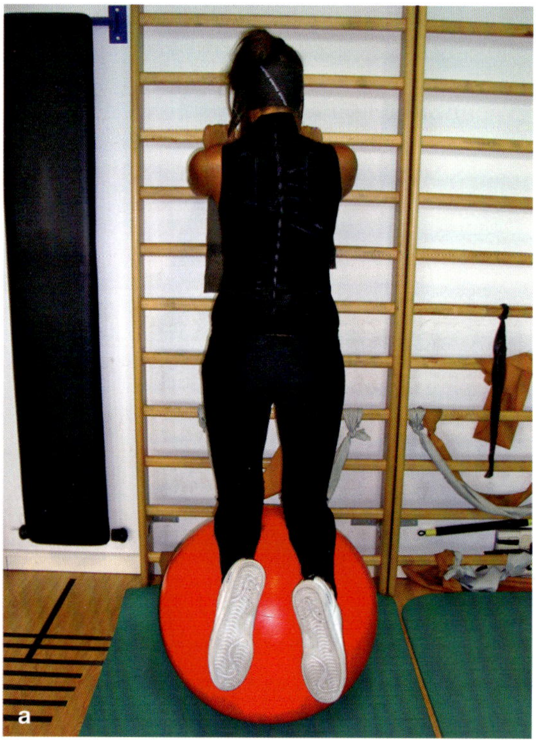

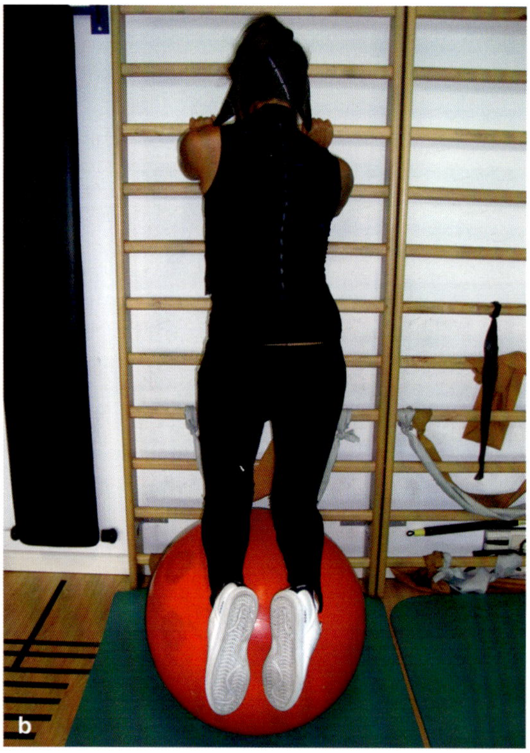

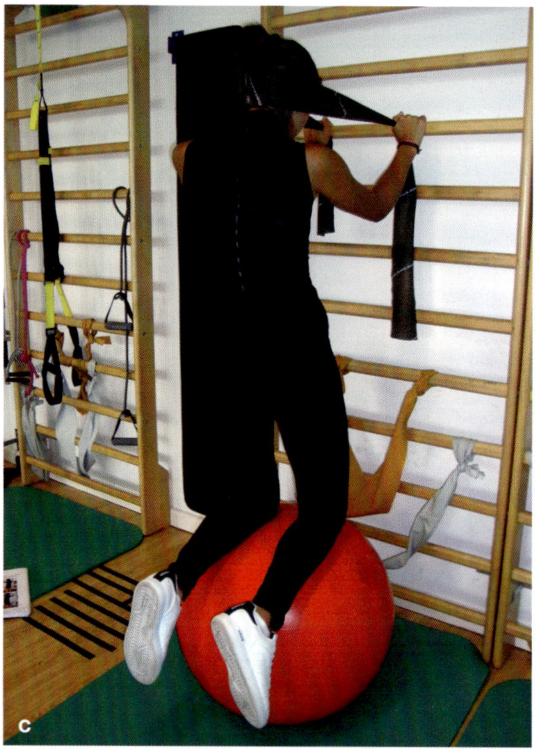

5

Structural Scoliosis, Dysmorphism, and Severe Dysmorphism

Group B

Group C

The exercises shown below may be integrated into the personalized rehabilitative protocol, under the supervision of the therapeutic work team.

We remind the reader that due to the complexity of the exercises proposed, and because of the required degree of consciousness of supports, proprioceptive stimulation, and corrections (even minimal ones), some exercises are only recommended for experienced patients (that is, patients who have practiced corrective exercises for a sufficient time and who have a developed consciousness of the exercises and of their own posture). Other patients may be slowly and progressively introduced to the proper execution of these exercises, gaining awareness and comprehension thereof.

Patients with structural scoliosis and significant dysmorphism are often prescribed a corrective orthopedic corset. The corset is also worn during the sessions of medical exercise and kinesiotherapy with elastic bands. Aerobic work in particular should be carried out in the corset.

The therapeutic path includes exercises that address:

- postural rehabilitation and balance reaction development
- gaining bodily awareness
- gaining awareness of defects
- self-correction
- strengthening
- stabilization
- coordinative ability development
- neuromotor integration development
- ergonomics
- respiratory training
- corrective asymmetrical exercises
- respiratory exercises with shaping
- relaxation techniques.

These types of exercises, although they have different objectives, should all be performed in parallel. The order in which the exercises are performed is not important as long as they are all performed, since they are all complementary and fundamental for structuring the corrective path. It is the task of the therapist following the patient to indicate amounts and types, as well as the order of execution or the time of introduction of new exercises into the protocol. This all necessarily depends on the patient's preparation, condition of muscular tone and trophism, physical training, and personal characteristics found during the kinesiological examination. For this reason we will avoid indicating specific quantities and numbers of repetitions of the exercises.

EXERCISE 5.1

Gaining Bodily Awareness

This is a self-correction exercise with emphasis on perception and awareness of the points of contact of the spine with the vertical bench. These are to be performed without the corset; the exercise is kyphotizing and corrective on a three-dimensional plane.

Execution - With the back resting against the wall, attention is paid to the perceived asymmetries of contact. After having taken awareness of this, the patient performs a deep inhalation and then initiates correction during exhalation, taking advantage of the elastic band (which passes behind the back at the dorsal hump). This exercise has three dimensions to its performance: kyphotization, lateralization, and derotation, bringing the upper limb homolateral to the concavity of the scoliotic curve into slight elevation compared to the contralateral one.

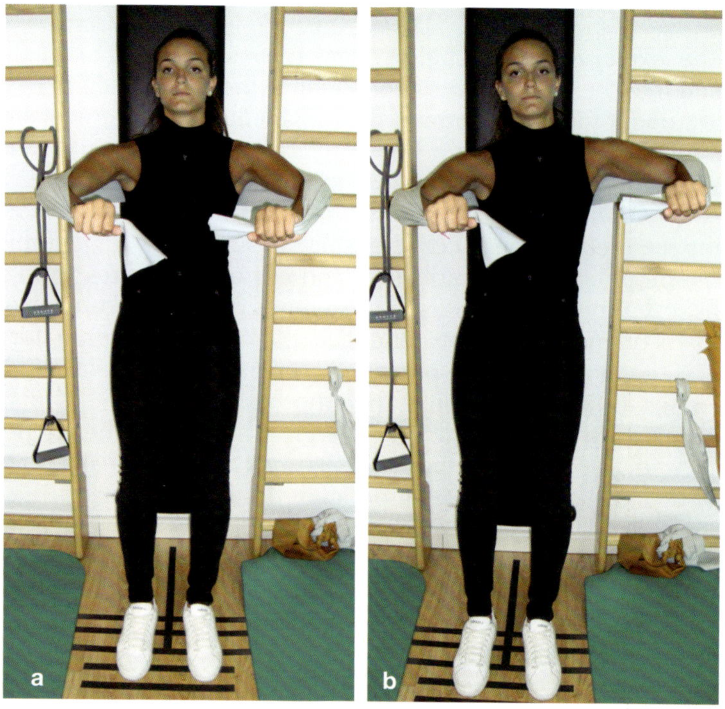

a, Starting position: awareness of contact;
b, three-dimensional correction.

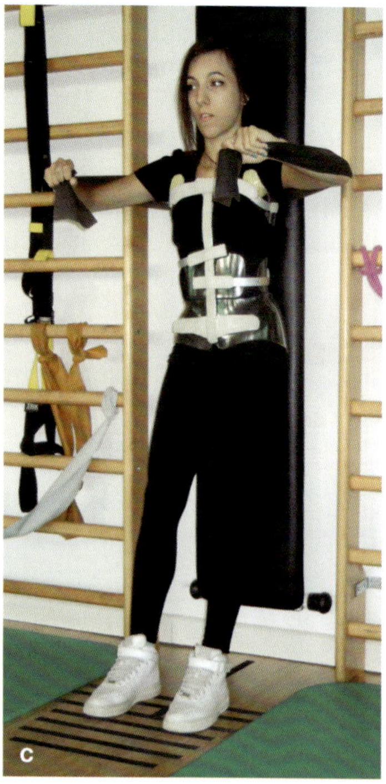

Variant - This exercise may also be performed while wearing the corset. Obviously, in this case, without the support of the elastic band on the hump (but rather on the corset), the sensations created by the corset pelota will be taken advantage of using the pelota itself and the arms as a corrective impulse.

EXERCISE 5.2

Gaining Awareness of Defects

This exercise is self-corrective and kyphotizing.

Execution - The patient is on the knees with the hands on the ground, and the elastic band around the back at the hump and held to the ground with the hands, which remain at shoulder level. The patient inhales against the elastic resistance; the patient kyphotizes the back and then exhales in a slow, prolonged manner, lateralizing and derotating the trunk.
Self-correction is performed with the use of the elastic band for a total of three corrective phases of kyphotization, lateralization, and derotation.

a, Starting position, with awareness of defects;
b, kyphotization;
c, lateralization and derotation.

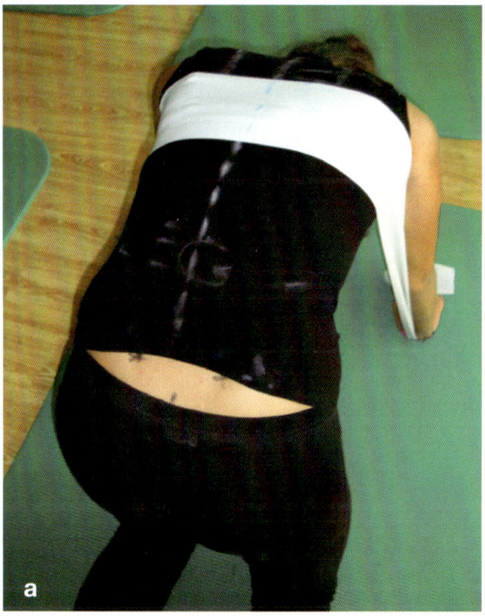
a

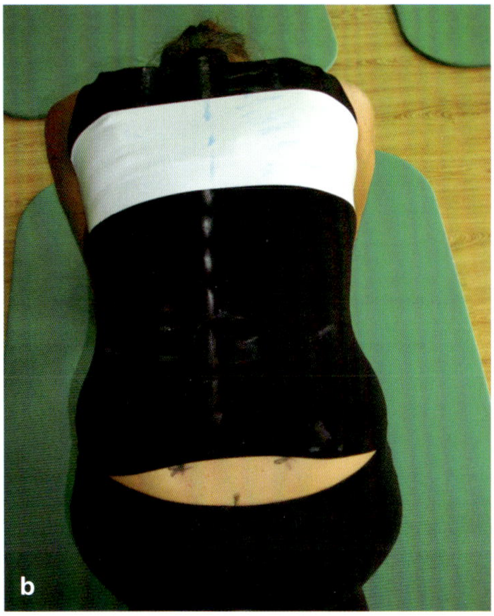
b

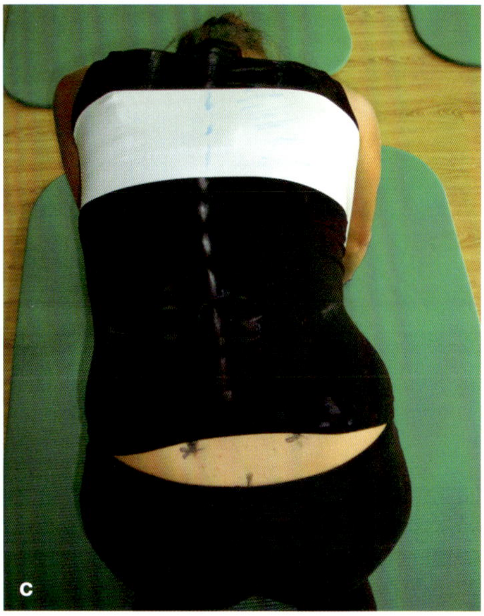
c

Group B

Group C

EXERCISE 5.3

Postural Rehabilitation and Self-correction

The objective of this exercise is postural correction and development of balance reactions.

Execution - The patient stands upright on the proprioceptive board. Correct posture and balance are sought with the use of the elastic band, which is positioned under the feet and held with the hands. This exercise may be performed while wearing the corset (**a**) or without it (**b**).

It is recommended that this exercise be performed in front of an orthopedic mirror in order to facilitate the gaining of consciousness of one's own posture.

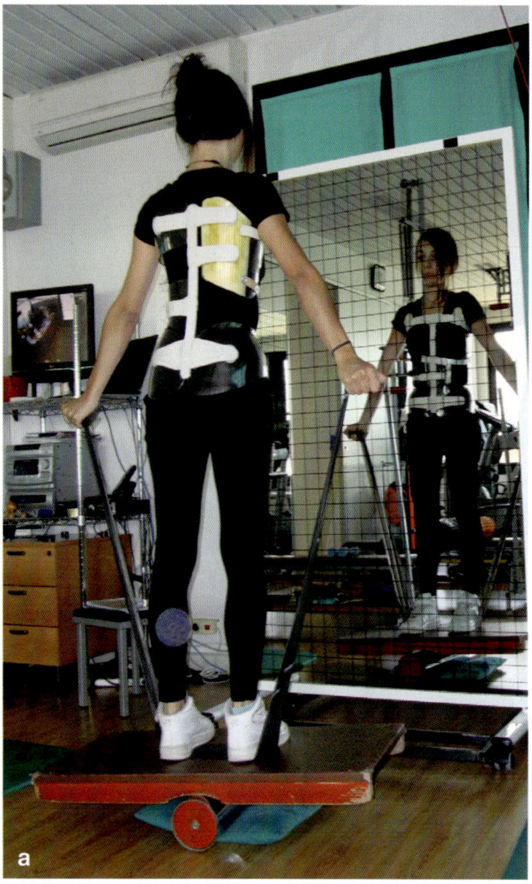

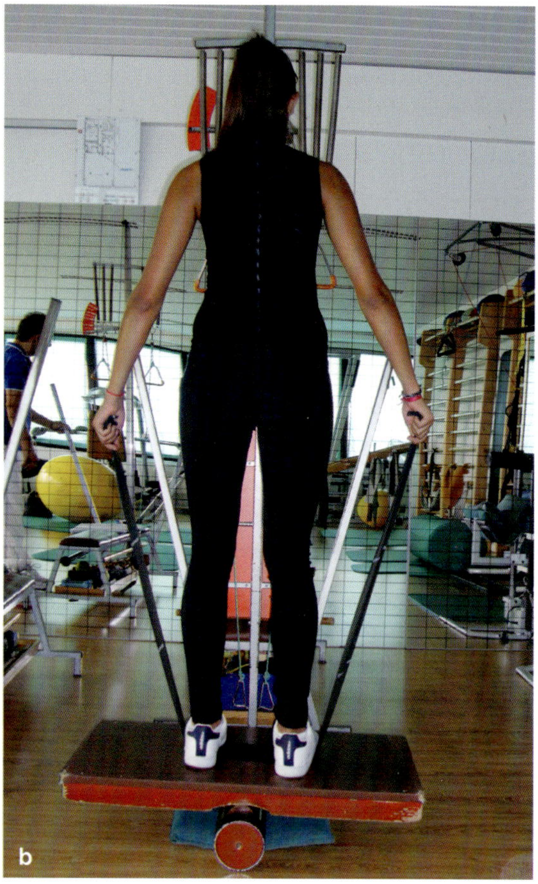

EXERCISE 5.4

Postural Rehabilitation

These exercises, performed while wearing the corset, refine postural reactions and develop balance reactions.

Execution - The patient is seated on the balance board, with the elastic band passing under the gluteus and both hands gripping the ends, ensuring to wrap the elbows with the elastic band. With arms at shoulder level, the patient raises the upper limbs laterally, maintaining balance (**a**, **b**) while gaining awareness and postural control via the mirror.

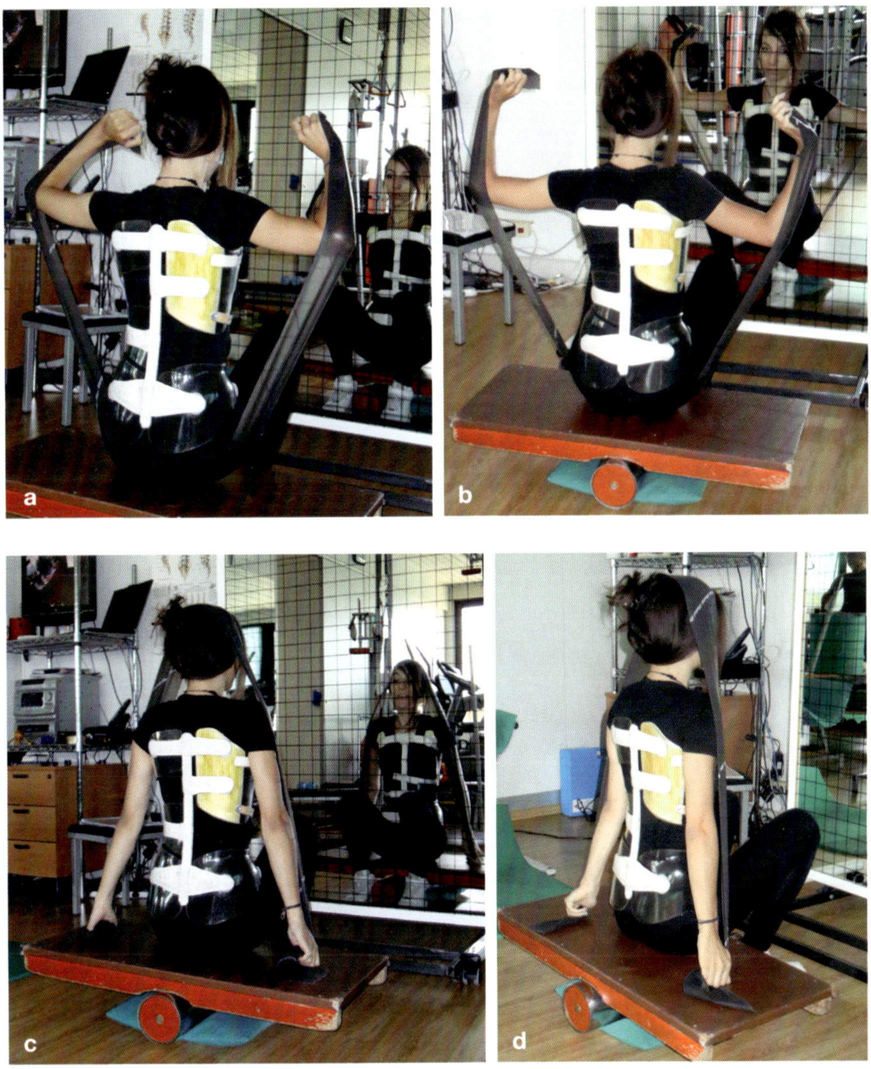

Variant - Seated on the balance board, wearing the corset, the elastic band is placed on the head and fixed to the balance board on both sides with the hands. The patient maintains extension "wriggling" out of the corset (**c**, **d**).

EXERCISE 5.5

Balance Reaction Development

The objective is the development of proprioceptive capabilities regarding balance and the muscles of the spine. The elastic band stimulates the proprioception of the muscles of the spine.

Execution - Patient is in quadruped position on a Swiss ball, with the elastic band around the back properly placed so as to wrap around the hump, with the ends of the band held by the hands, which rest on the ball. The patient performs postural self-control, in search of balance and its maintenance. Once balance is reached, the three-dimensional correction parameters are implemented (kyphotization, lateralization, derotation).

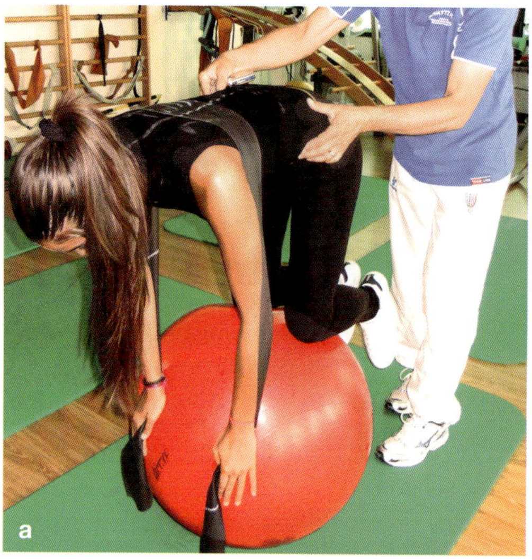

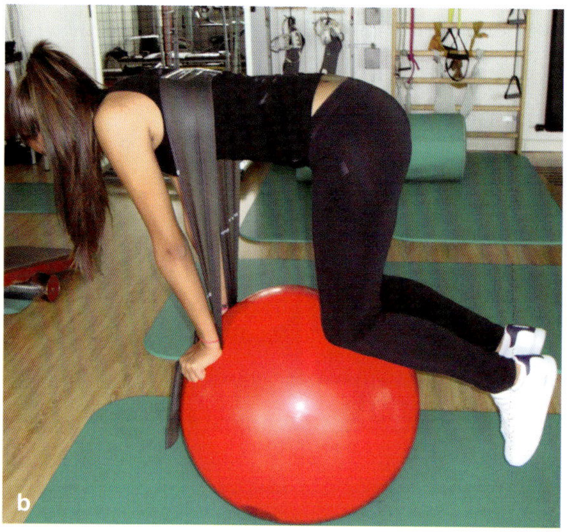

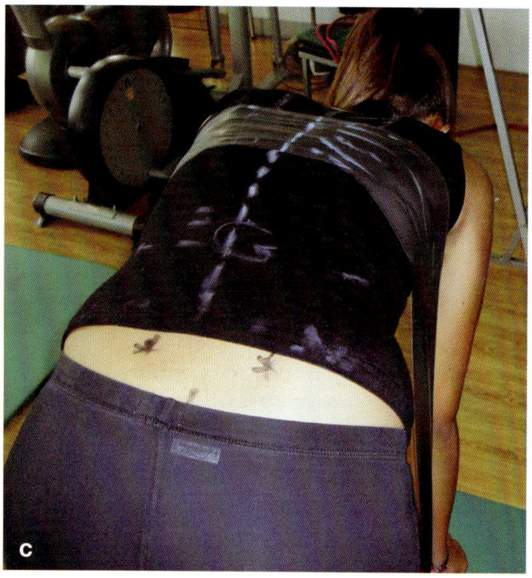

a, Preparation of exercise, search for balance;
b, maintenance of balance and kyphotization;
c, lateralization (to the left) and light derotation in a counter-clockwise direction.

EXERCISE 5.6

Self-correction

The objective is to gain consciousness of defects and self-correction in the three dimensions: kyphotization, lateralization, derotation.

Execution - The patient holds the elastic band with the hands (arms forward) and induces greater tension from the side of the convexity of the dorsal curve. While positioning the elastic band, care must be taken to "wrap around" the dorsal hump and keep the elbows within it. Destablization is induced by flexing the lower limbs and lifting the body with the feet, keeping the trunk flexed by 30 degrees.
Self-correction is initiated with the three phases in this order: kyphotization (**a**), lateralization, and derotation (**b**).

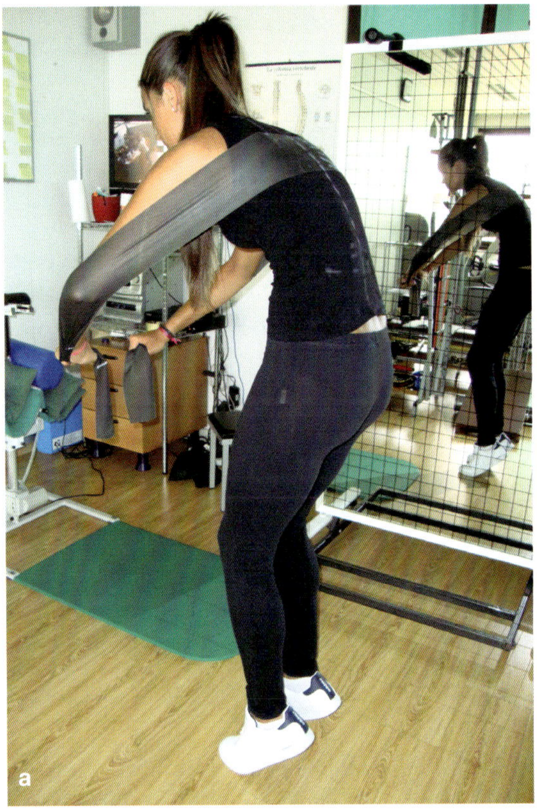
a

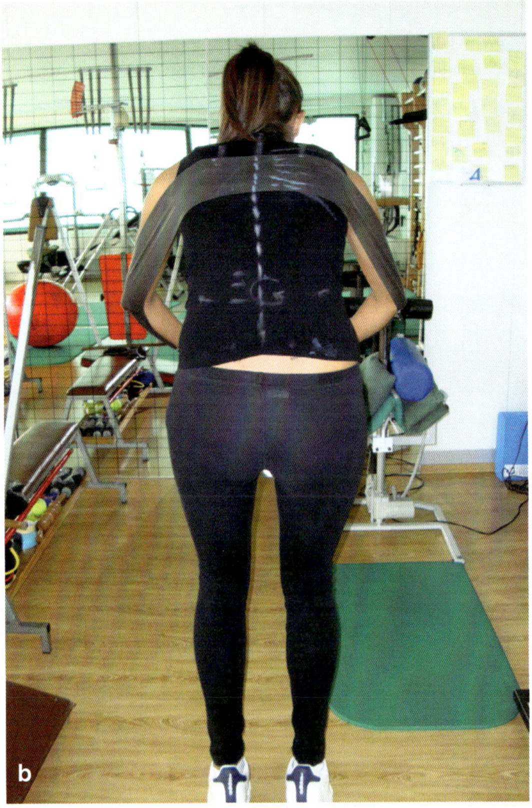
b

EXERCISE 5.7

Decompensated Stretching with Three-dimensional Correction

The goal of this exercise is the correction of the scoliotic curve (kyphotization, lateralization and derotation) simultaneously with the stretching of the anti-gravitational posterior chain.

Execution - The patient is seated in front of the wall bars with an elastic band hooked onto a rung and held in tension by the feet (stretching the lower limbs). The patient holds a second elastic band in tension, which is passed around another, higher rung of the wall bars (above the patient's head) while correction exercises are performed.

While keeping the two elastic bands in tension, the patient performs the three corrections of the scoliotic curve: first kyphotization, then lateralization and derotation. An optional support placed under the left gluteus (in cases of right lumbar curvature) helps to neutralize the right lumbar compensatory curve. A cushion under the feet simply facilitates the sliding of the feet for keeping the elastic band in tension.

a, Starting position;
b, extension of the lower limbs and traction with the upper limbs; kyphotization;
c, lateralization and derotation.

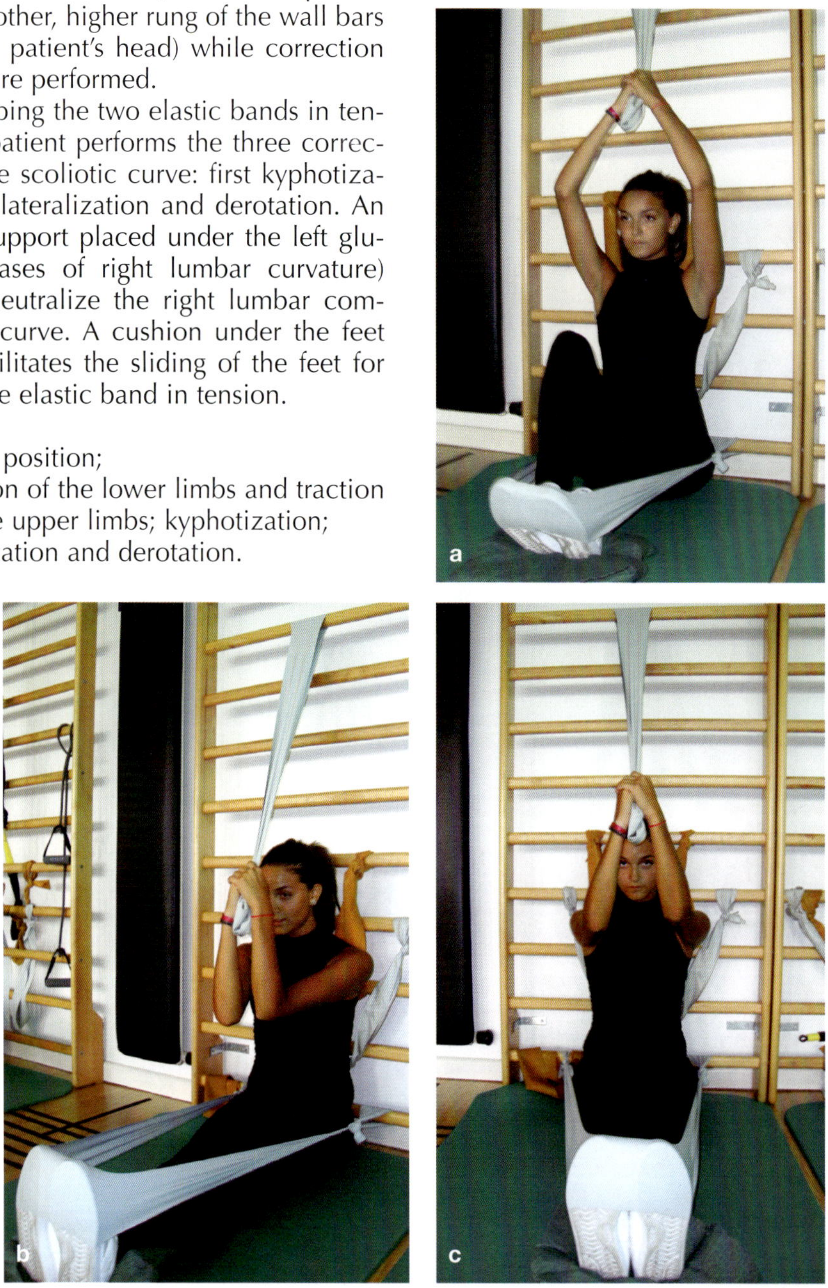

EXERCISE 5.8

Self-correction

This exercise is corrective and kyphotizing (to be performed without the corset).

Execution - The elastic band wraps around the head and the nape of the neck and is held between the hands, which are gripped to the wall bars in front of the patient. The patient sits on a Swiss ball and performs three-dimensional correction of the back with retroposition of the trunk and the neck, keeping the head in place with isometric contraction. This exercise is performed in two phases:

- isometric contraction, briefly inhaling
- correction during slow and prolonged exhalation.

The right lower limb is brought backwards in order to maintain balance with lumbar compensation. Self-correction is performed during exhalation, totaling three processes: kyphotization, lateralization, and derotation.

a, Preparation of the exercise and kyphotization;
b, lateralization;
c, derotation and three-dimensional correction.

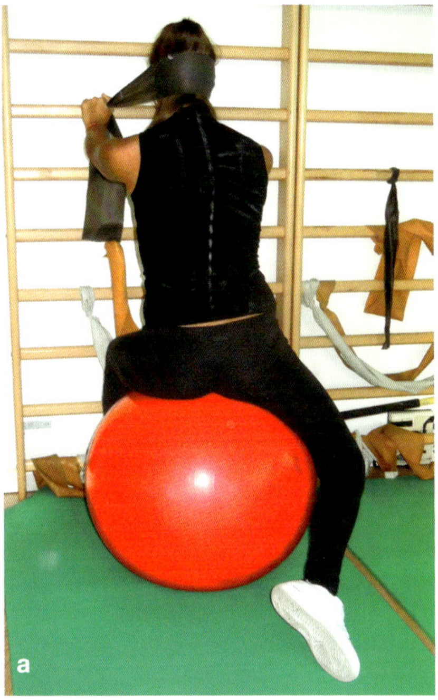
a

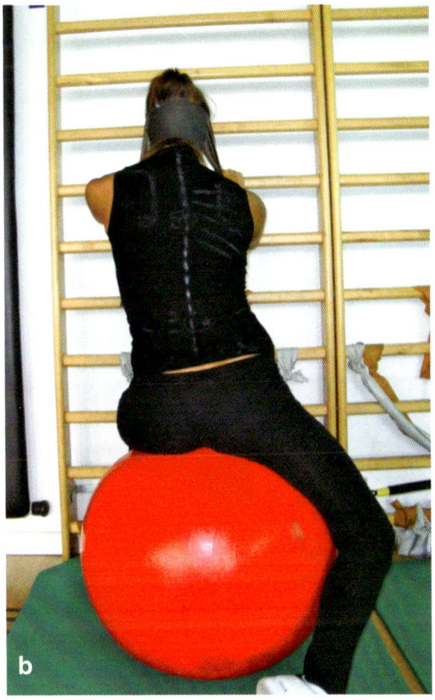
b

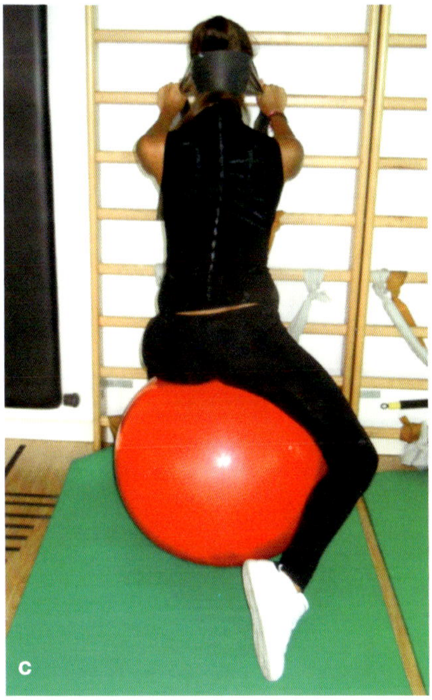
c

Group B

Group C

EXERCISE 5.9

Self-correction with Corset

This exercise, similar to the preceding one, is corrective and kyphotizing, and is performed with the corset.

Execution - Patient is seated on a Swiss ball in front of the walls bar, the right foot (in cases of left secondary lumbar curvature) slightly raised off the ground, with the elastic band passed around the head (the ends are held by the hands, which rest on the wall bars). The patient performs three-dimensional correction of the back with retroposition of the trunk and the neck, keeping the head in place with isometric contraction. The correction is done during slow, prolonged exhalation, and consists, as usual, of the sum of the three corrective phases of kyphotization, lateralization, and derotation.

a, Starting position, with right foot raised by one peg to correct the lumbar compensatory curve;
b, kyphotization with retraction of the head (slight kyphotization of the dorsal spine);
c, three-dimensional correction.

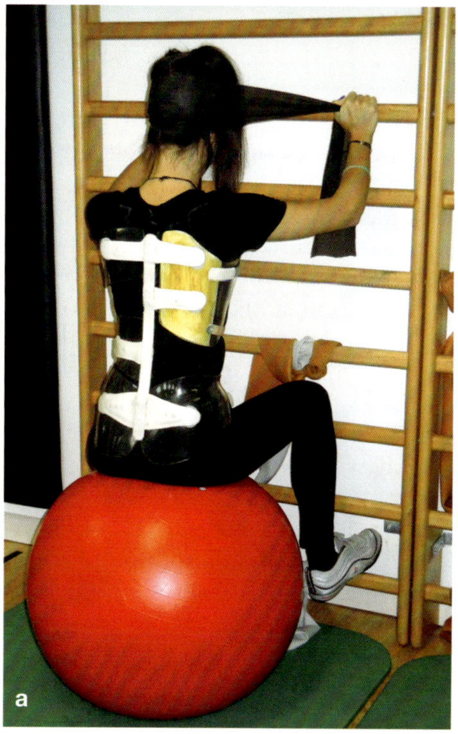

a

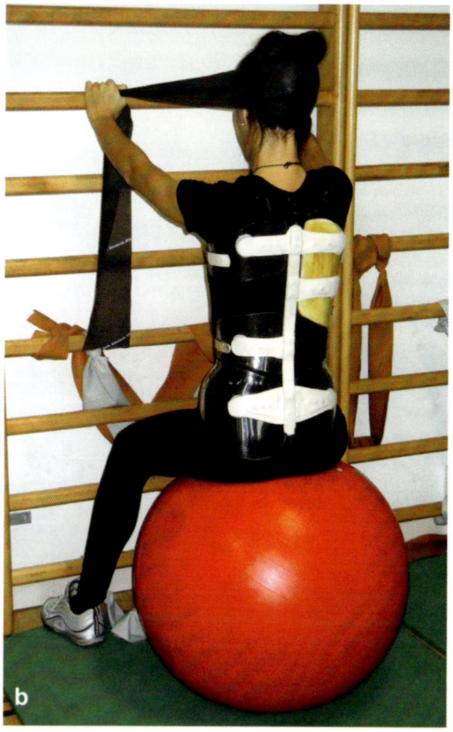

b

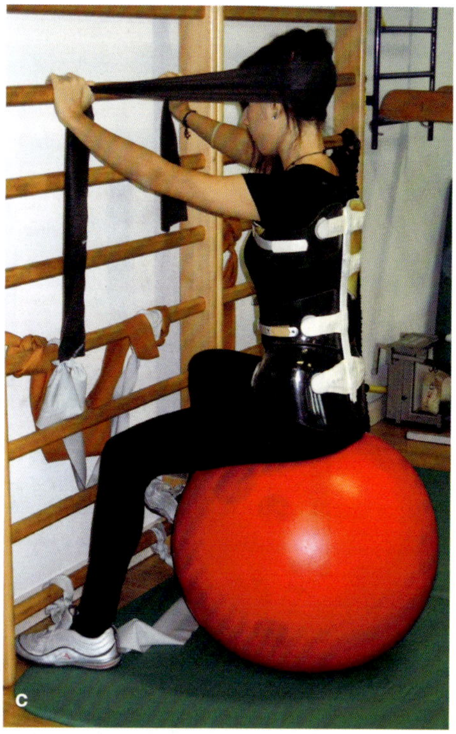

c

EXERCISE 5.10

Self-correction

This is a kyphotizing exercise with correction due to the pressure of the elastic band.

Execution - Patient is on the ground, in the prone position, with the arms in candlestick position, and the elastic band wrapping around the area of interest (dorsal hump). A cylindrical cushion under the abdomen avoids "hyperlordosization" (assuming a position of hyperlordosis). A tennis ball in the left hand provides an action that can facilitate correction (from the side of the concavity of the curve). In the first phase of the exercise, the patient inhales, then exhales slowly (the back is kyphotized during this step); then, squeezing the ball, kyphotization, lateralization, and derotation are performed from the same side (three-dimensional correction).

a, Preparation of the exercise;
b, kyphotization and lateralization;
c, overall view with the three phases of self-correction.

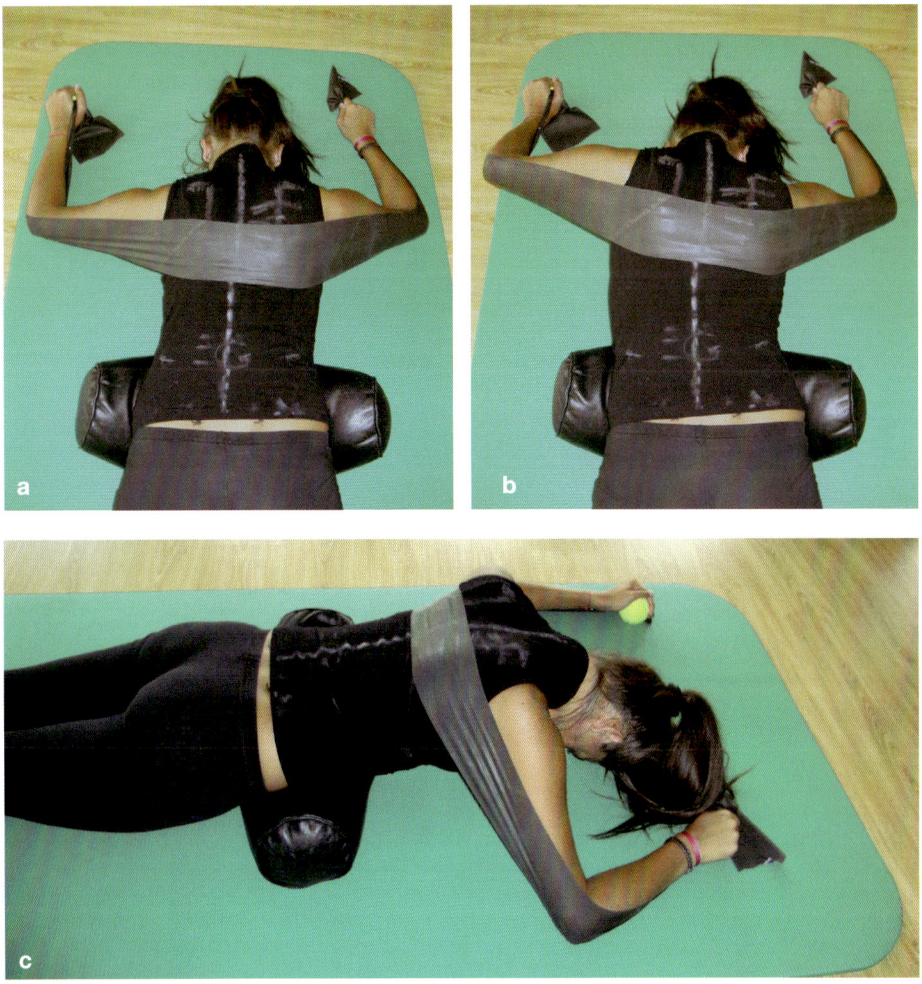

EXERCISE 5.11

Self-correction

This is a three-dimensional correction of the dorsal curve with traction of the elastic band.

Execution - This exercise is similar to the previous one. The patient assumes the candlestick position (**a**), but in this case there is a forced lateralization by the single-handed grasping of the elastic band (both ends to the left), which allows an increase in the tension-traction force, sensitizing the direction of the correction (in the case of scoliosis with right primary curvature, lateralization is needed to the left, as indicated by the arrow; **b**).

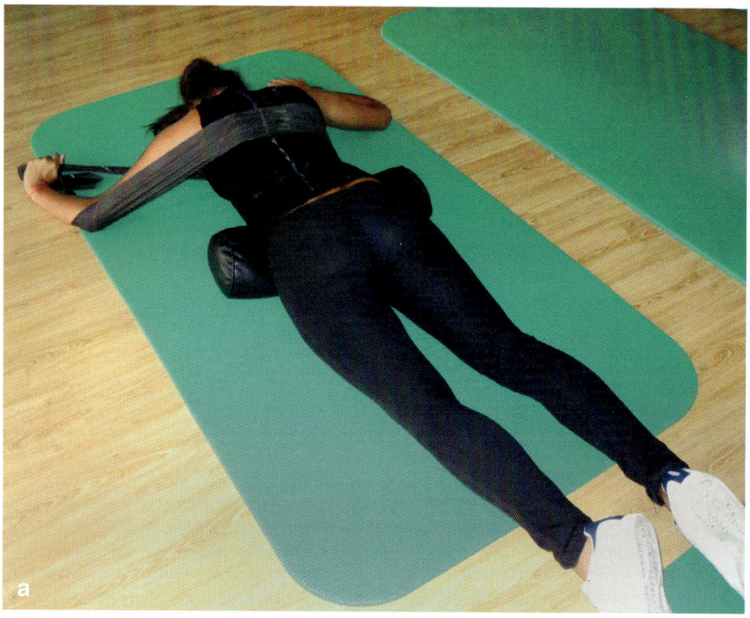

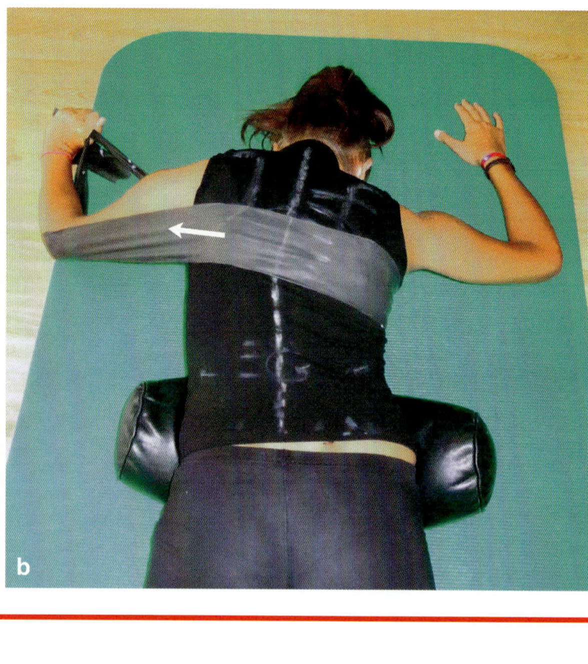

EXERCISE 5.12

Self-correction, Facilitating (with Corset)

This is a three-dimensional correction of the dorsal curve.

Execution - Patient is in the supine position, with the knees raised. The elastic band is used to cover the dorsal area and the upper limbs, ensuring to keep the elbow within it. In the exhalation phase, attention is paid to the perception of variations via the principles of the correction on the three planes of space, keeping a fixed point with the upper limbs. Patients wearing corsets must learn to perceive corrections, even minimal ones, through the corset pelota and not the elastic band on the hump.

a, **b**, **c**, execution with the corset, seen from three points of observation; in c, the force with greater resistance performed with the left upper limb can be seen;

d, execution without corset: seeking correction on the three planes of space.

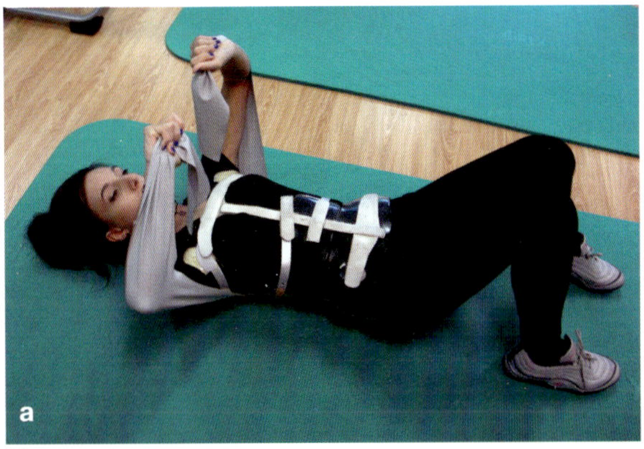

a

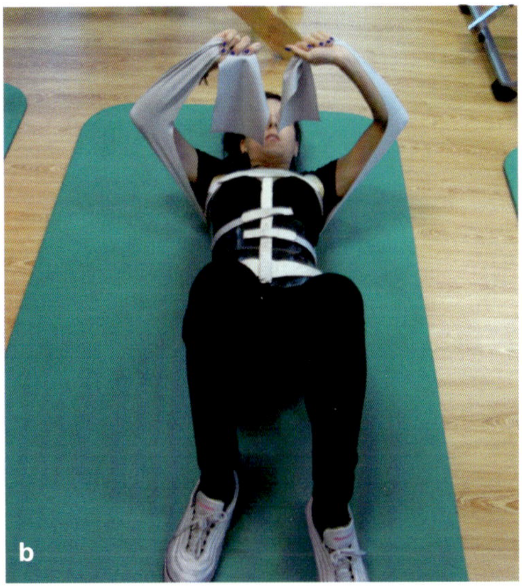

b

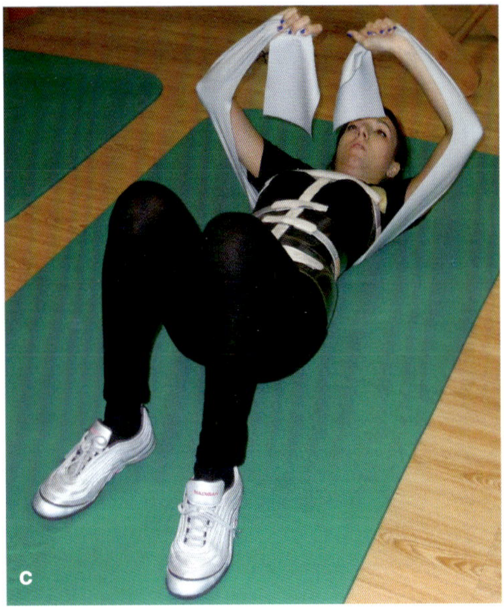

c

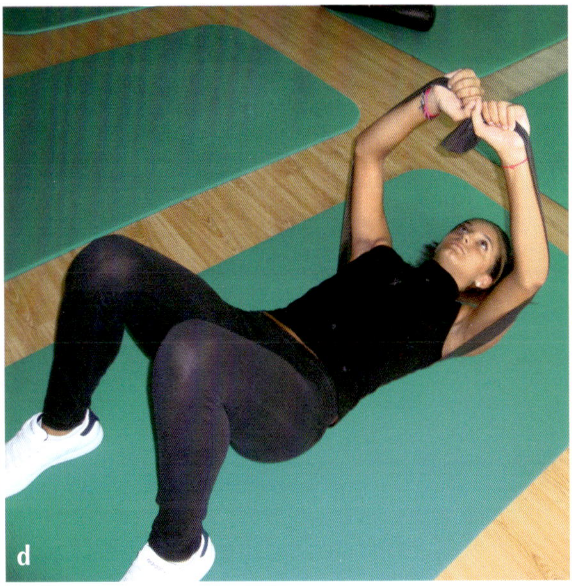

d

Group B

Group C

EXERCISE 5.13

Self-correction

This is a three-dimensional correction and kyphotizing exercise.

Execution - The exercise is carried out with a corset. The convex ladder is resting on its first rungs. The patient, while inhaling, pulls the elastic band (which is fixed to the wall bars below the convex ladder) in the direction of the pubis (**a**). The forehead is supported on the ladder. During exhalation, the patient kyphotizes, lateralizes, and derotates the spine from the side opposite to the dorsal pelota in order to complete the three-dimensional correction (**b**). If necessary, light traction of the lower limb toward the head may be performed through contact with the dorsum of the foot (from the side of the concavity of the lumbar compensatory curve; **c**).

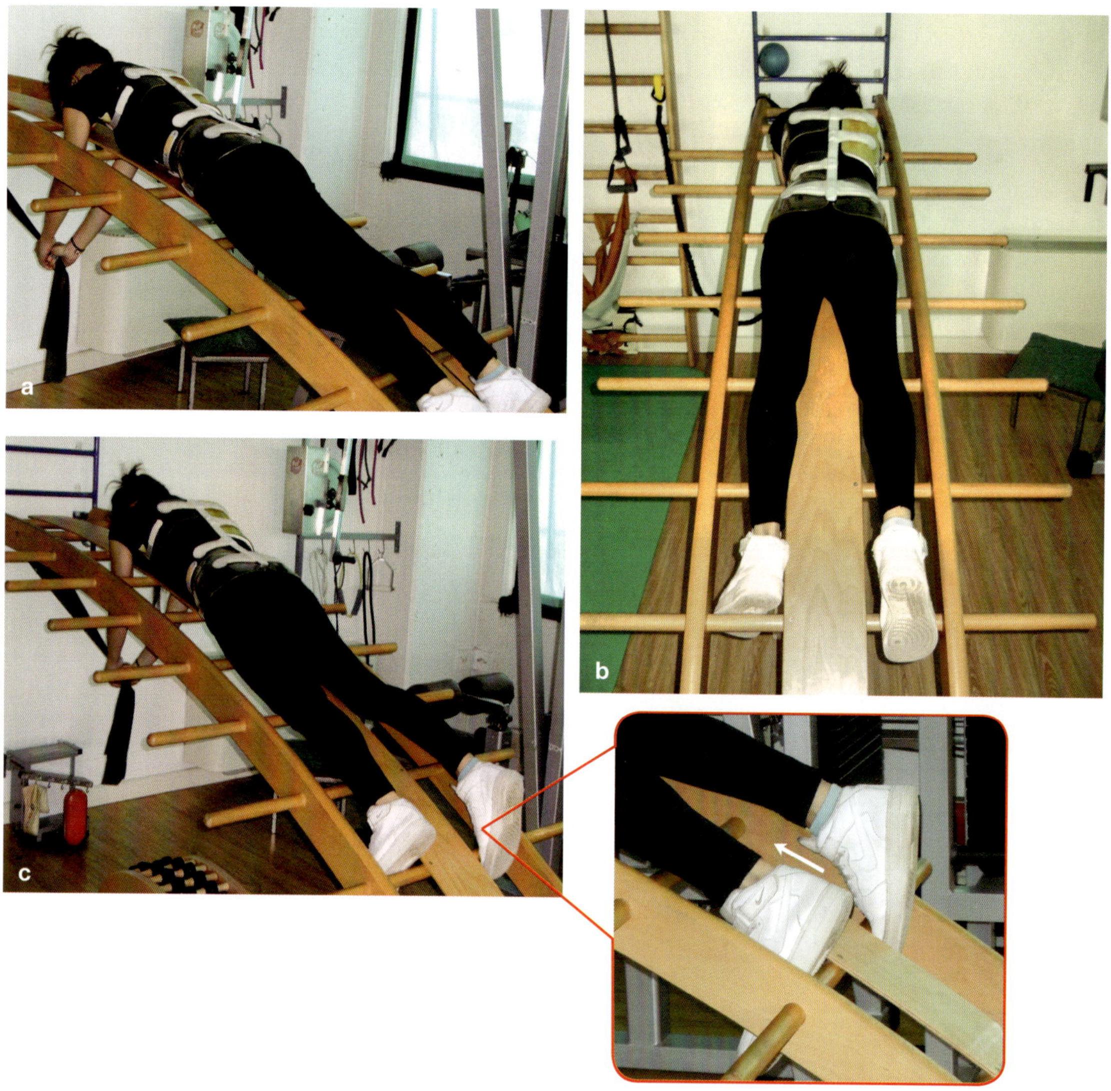

The previous exercise may also be performed without the corset. The cushion or roller under the abdomen may be useful to facilitate support (**d**). Kyphotization, pivoting isometrically on the arms, then lateralization and derotation (**e**).
Close-up view, with the corrective movement well-executed. The drawing of the hump with chalk facilitates the reading of the correction made (**f**).

Group B

Group C

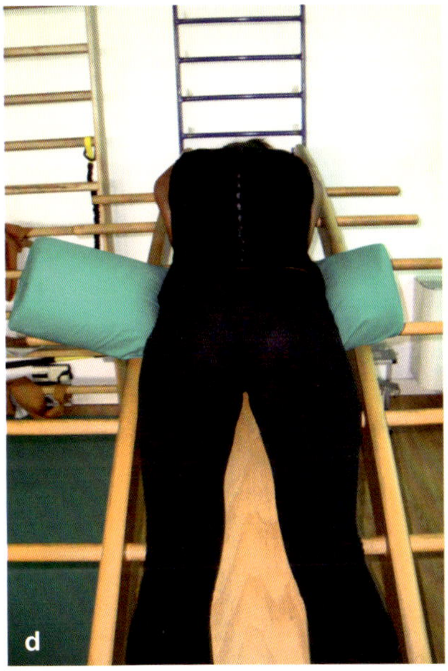

d

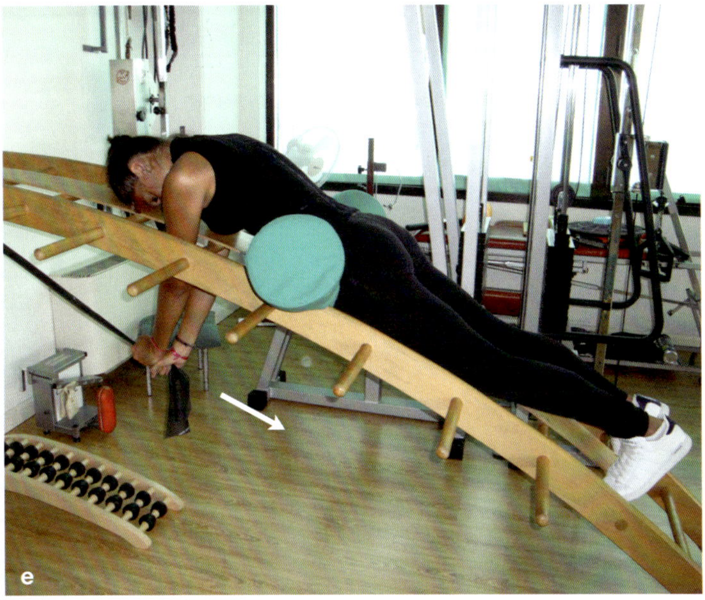

e

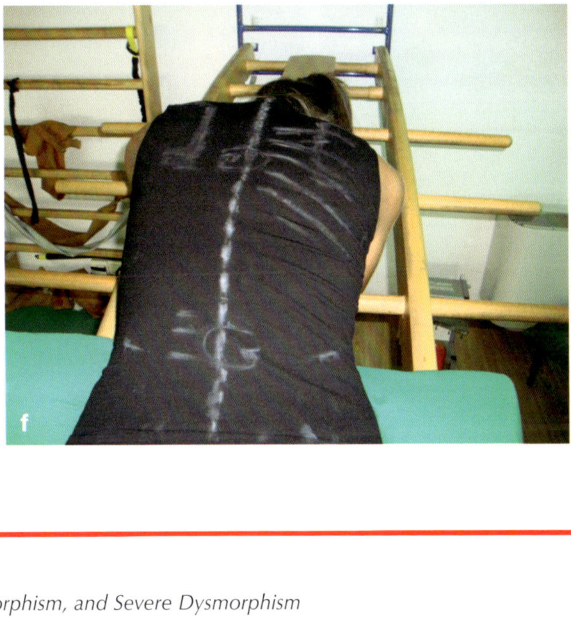

f

EXERCISE 5.14

Non-compensated Stretching and Correction

This exercise provides non-compensated stretching with self-induced elongation and correction of the dorsal hump.

Execution - In a state of non-compensated elongation of the posterior chain, kyphotization is sought after the patient has inhaled, pivoting on the elastic with the hands (**a**). Next, the three-dimensional correction of the dorsal hump is sought during exhalation, having the elastic initially slide to obtain a lifting of the upper limb (the one corresponding to the concavity of the curve); then, a tension-traction force is made with the same arm, which induces lateralization and derotation and completes the three-dimensional correction (**b**). The cushion under the feet has the simple function of facilitating the sliding of the feet over the mat.

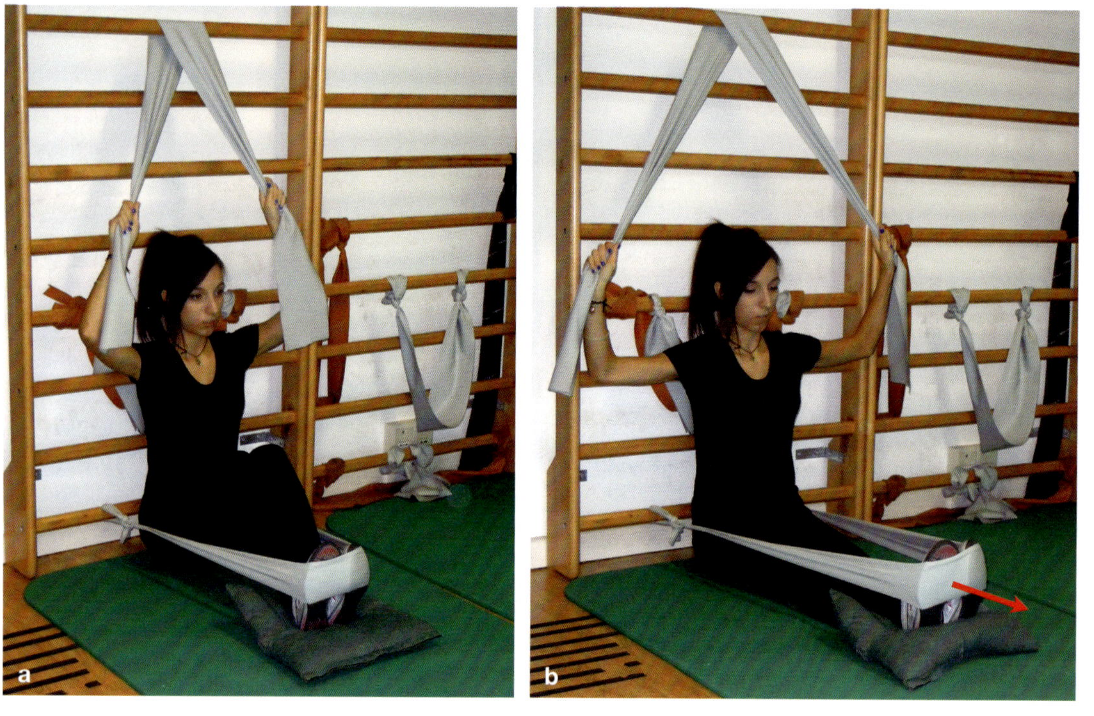

EXERCISE 5.15

Muscular Strengthening

This is an exercise for general strengthening and strengthening of the lower limbs.

Execution - The patient is in the supine position: the lower limbs are brought together at right angles, then the legs are alternatingly bent and stretched against the resistance of the elastic (**a**). This exercise may be performed both with (**b**) and without the corset (**c**).

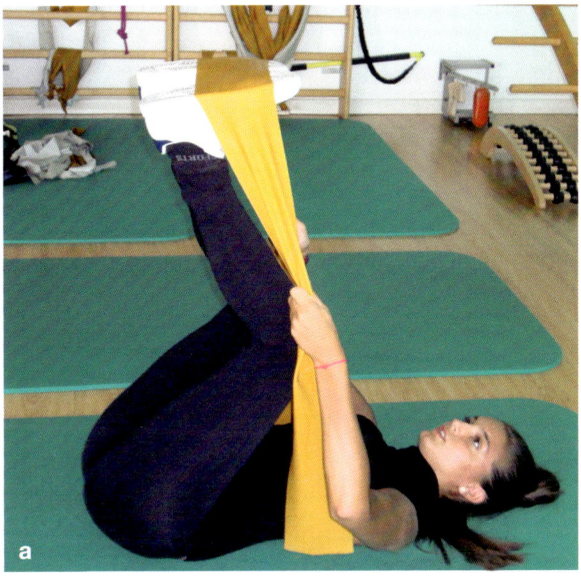

a

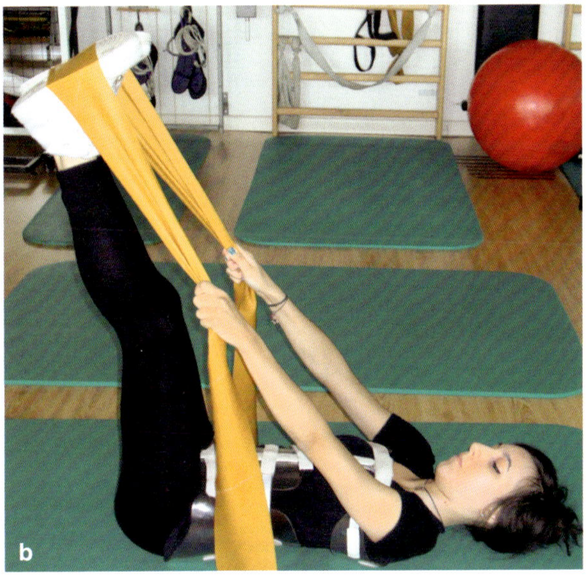

b

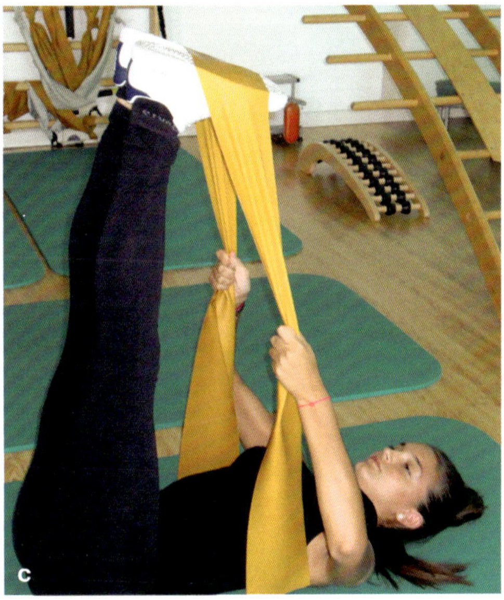

c

Group B

Group C

EXERCISE 5.16

Muscular Strengthening

This provides strengthening of the abdominal muscles with dorsal and lumbar correction.

Execution - The patient lies in front of the wall bars, with the lower limbs raised and a medicine ball between the knees: the patient pulls the elastic (which is fixed on the wall bars above the head) toward the knees, keeping the abdominal muscles isometrically in tension. Pivoting on the elastic, the patient corrects the dorsal scoliotic curve in three dimensions during exhalation. The knees hold the 1 kg medicine ball and rotate with the pelvis from the part opposite the lumbar pelota in order to reduce compensation. This exercise may be done with (**a**-**c**) and without the corset (**d**, **e**).

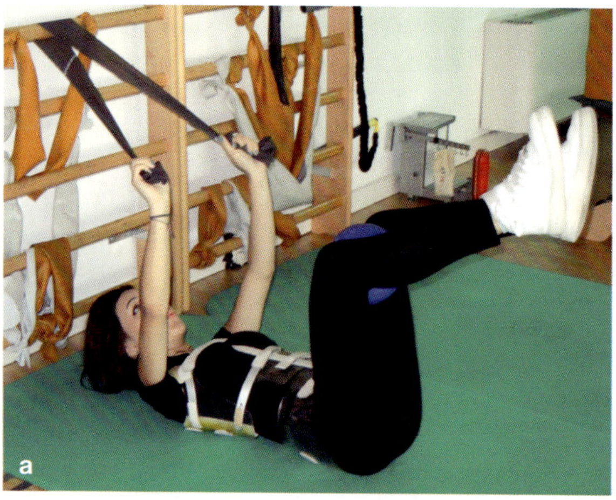

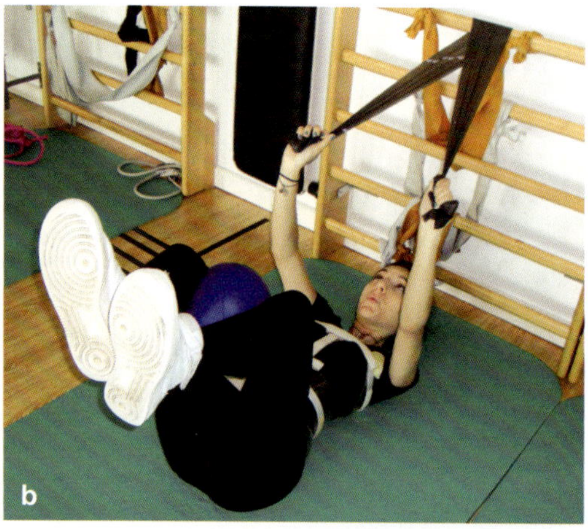

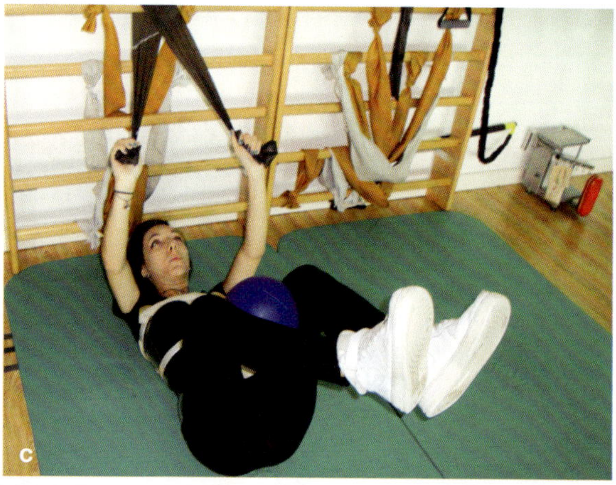

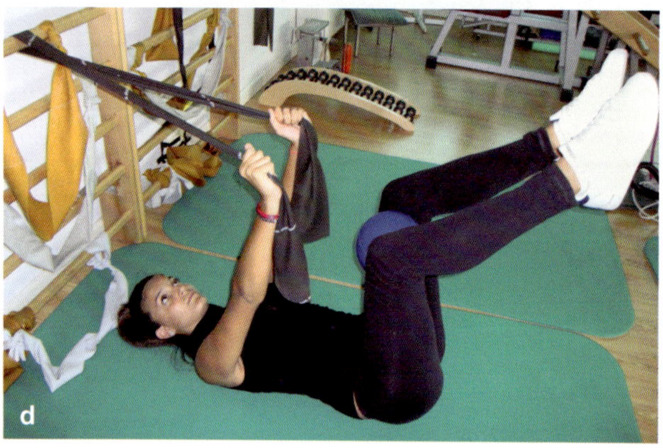

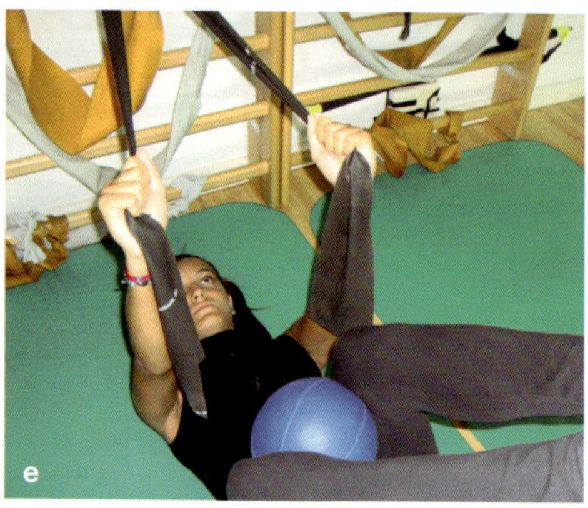

EXERCISE 5.17

Kyphotizing Corrective Exercise

Self-correction of the scoliotic curve. This exercise is kyphotizing, and corrective for the back during exhalation.

Execution - The patient is seated on a Swiss ball for greater correction of lumbar compensation; the elastic band is fixed to the wall bars with both extremities. The elastic is gripped with the elbows wrapped, and the elastic is pulled outward, seeking kyphotization, lateralization, and derotation in the direction of the correction. This exercise may be performed while not wearing the corset (**a**) or while wearing it (**b**).
An additional correction of the lumbar compensation may occur via the retroposition of the right lower limb (**d**).

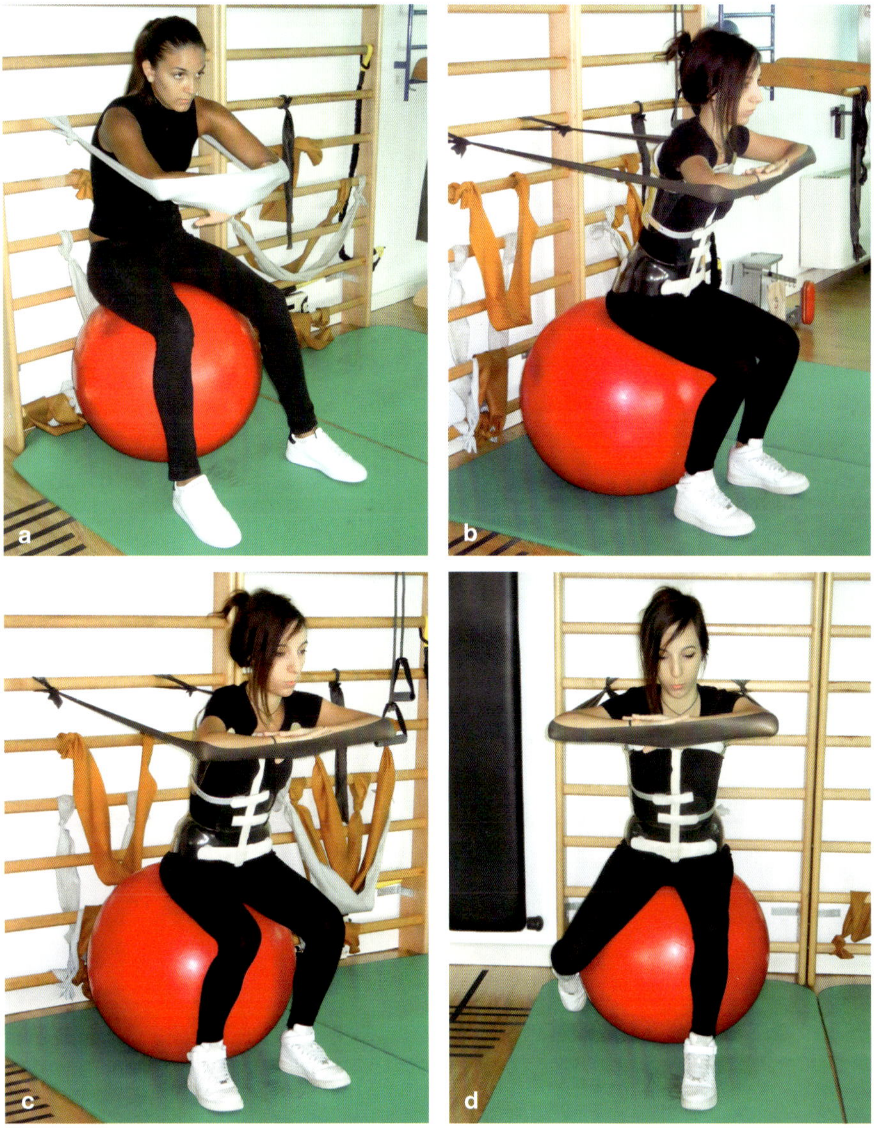

Group B

Group C

EXERCISE 5.18

Muscular Strengthening/corrective

The objective of this exercise is the strengthening of the paravertebral muscles with three-dimensional correction.

Execution - The patient is seated on a Swiss ball, positioned exactly over the vertical projection of the "Magri turtle", which is hooked onto the wall bars at the ideal height for the patient. The ends of the elastic band are tied to the wall bars; the elastic is gripped, leaving the elbows wrapped, and the elastic is pulled outward. The patient pushes with the head toward the "turtle", seeking a fixed point for the purposes of correction and strengthening of the paravertebral muscles.

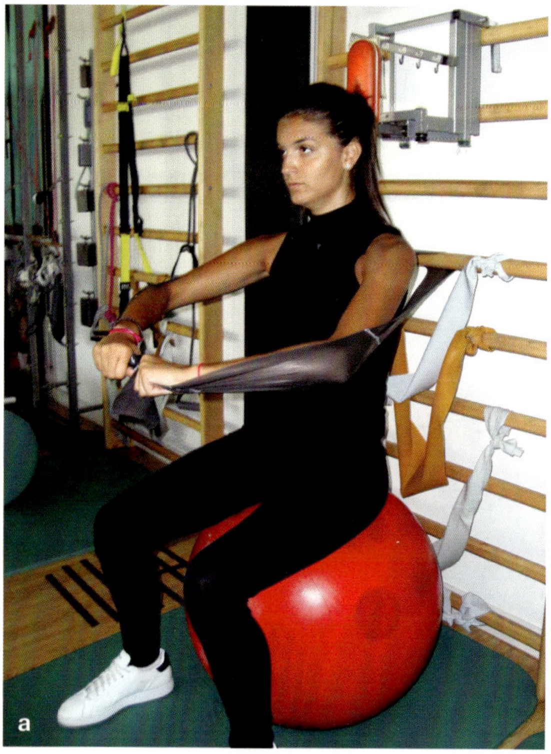

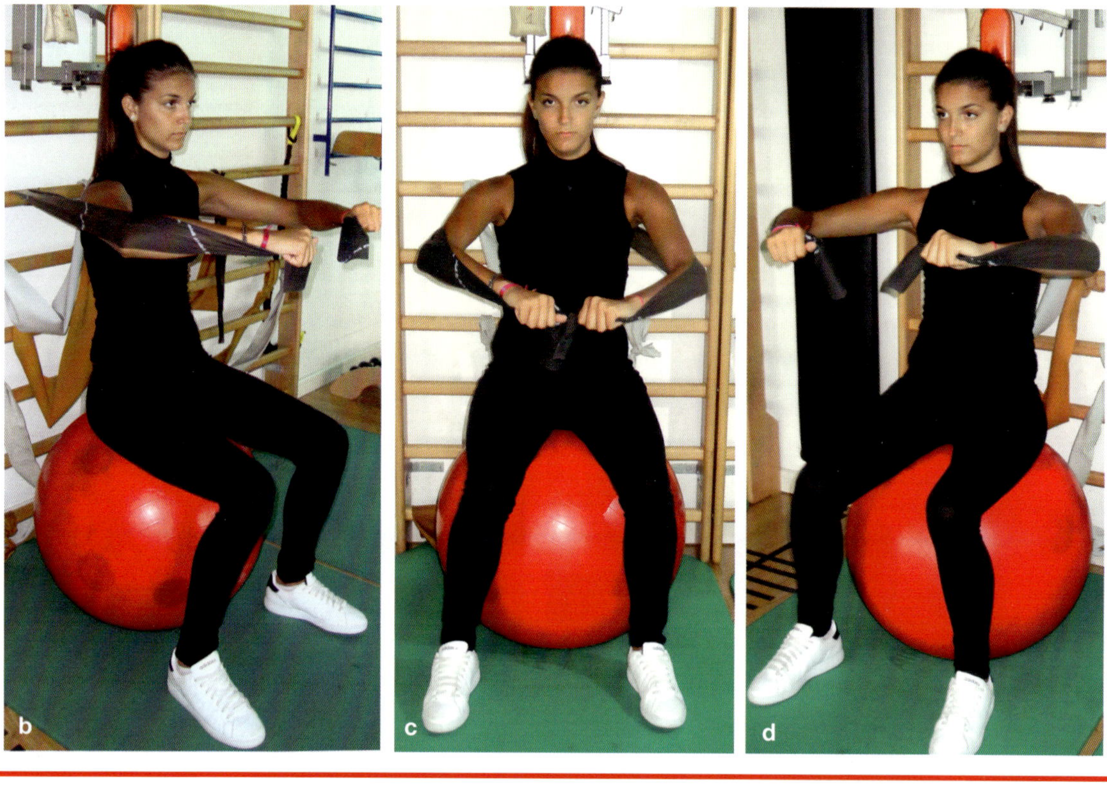

Variant - Same position and same exercise for patients with the corset. The corrections achieved are integrated in this exercise.
A stool could also be used for the seat, but the ball is recommended for the possibility of correcting the lumbar compensation due to the retroposition of one leg (**f**).

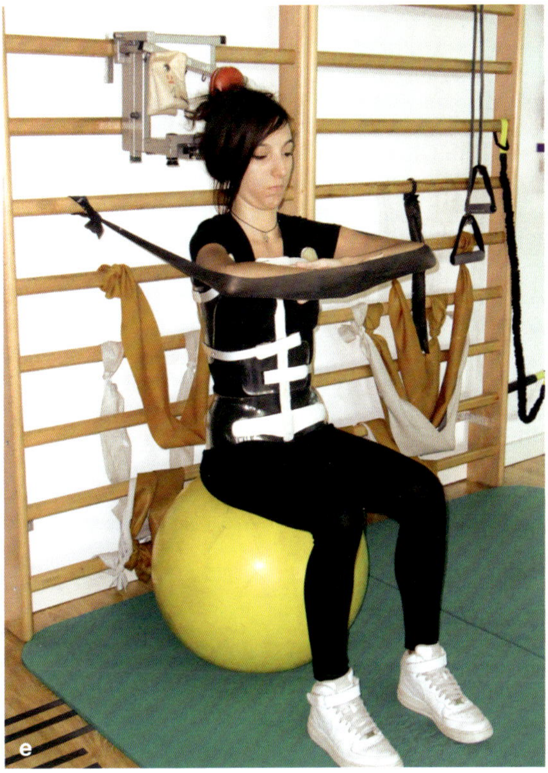

e

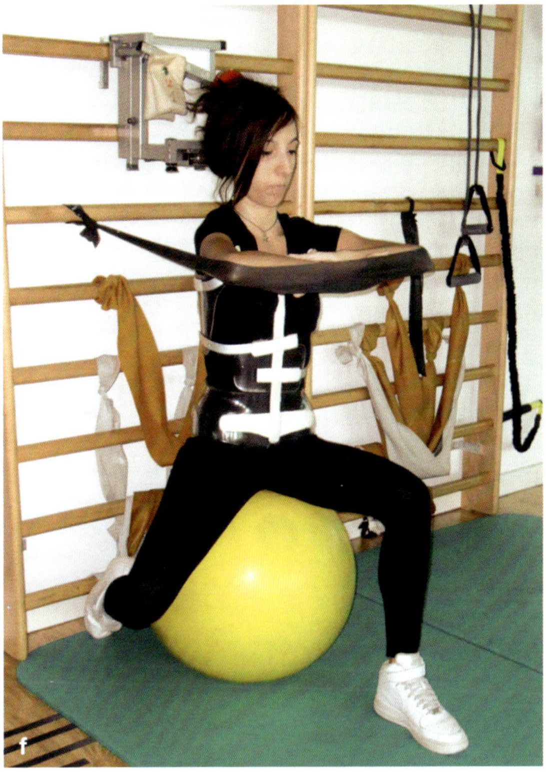

f

The Magri turtle: The device used was conceived by my friend and colleague, Professor Magri, and is commonly called "the Magri turtle". It hooks easily onto the wall bars at the proper height and allows the patient to perform self-stretching with strengthening of the paravertebral muscles. In addition to self-stretching, in this case it is used as a fixed point to perform/facilitate the corrections required on the three planes of space.

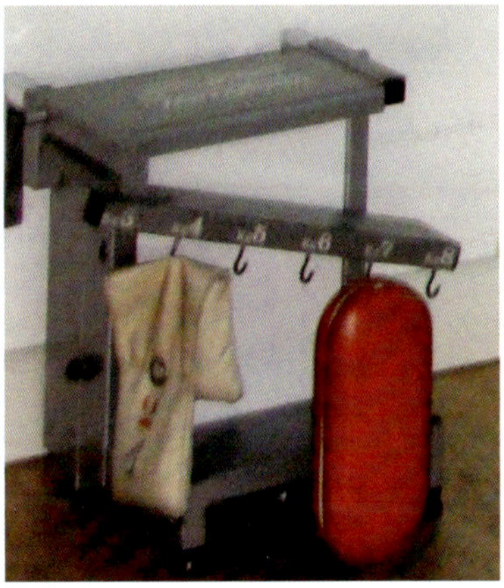

EXERCISE 5.19

Muscular Strengthening/corrective
The objective of this exercise is the strengthening of the paravertebral muscles and three-dimensional correction.

Execution - The patient is seated on a stool positioned exactly over the vertical projection of the "Magri turtle", which is hooked onto the wall bars at the ideal height for the patient. An elastic band, the ends of which are fixed to the wall bars, is placed over the chest. This elastic band has both ends on the left side to facilitate the correction of a right dorsal hump. The arm, holding a second elastic band with less intensity than the first, pulls on it in order to exert a traction on the dorsal hump. Three-dimensional correction is promoted by the elastic bands by pushing on the "turtle" with the head (**a-e**).

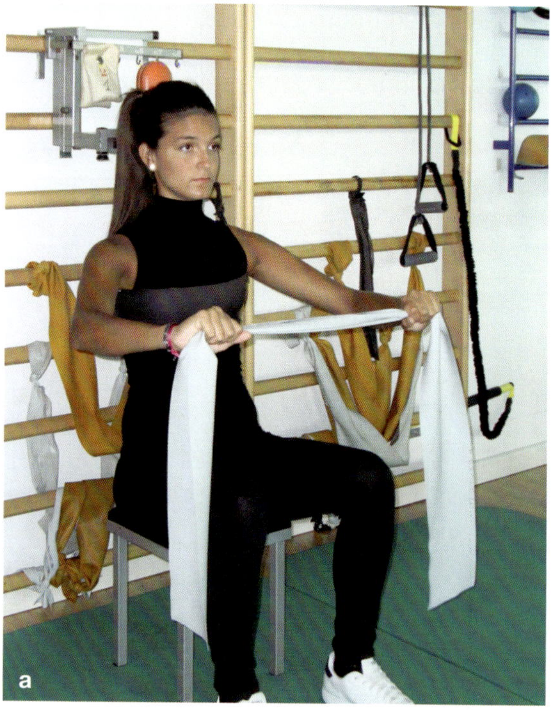
a

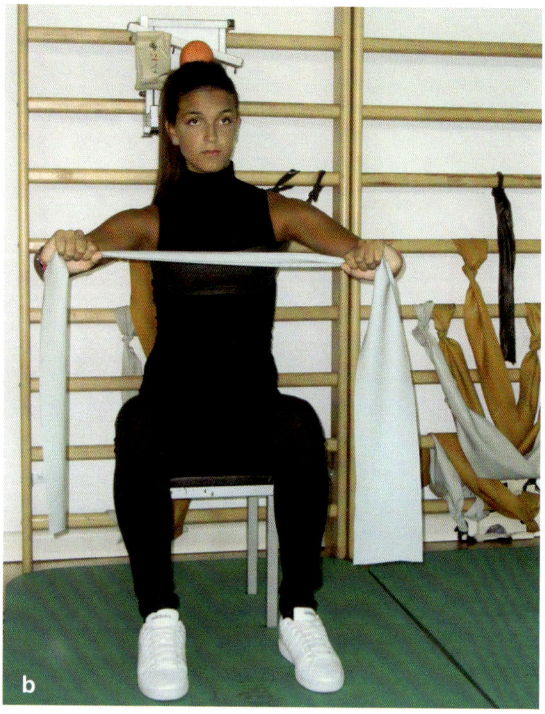
b

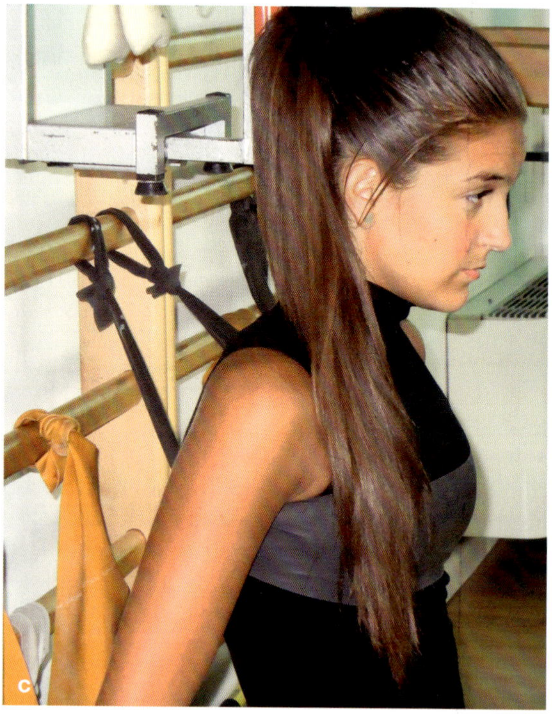
c

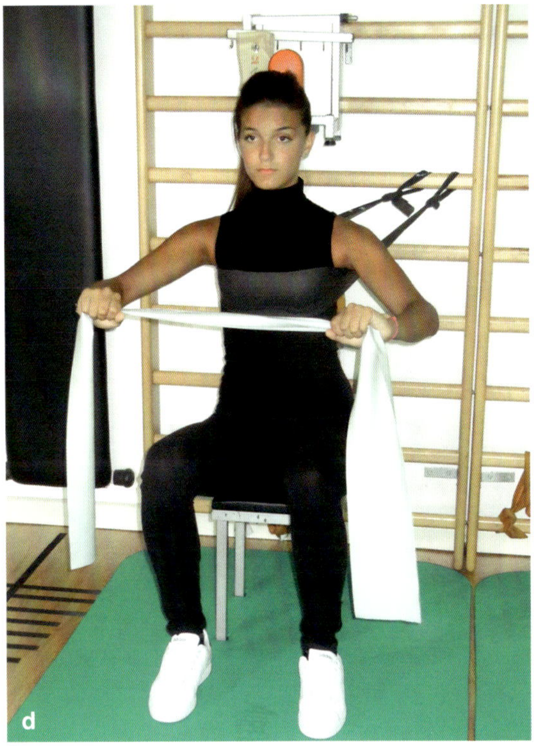

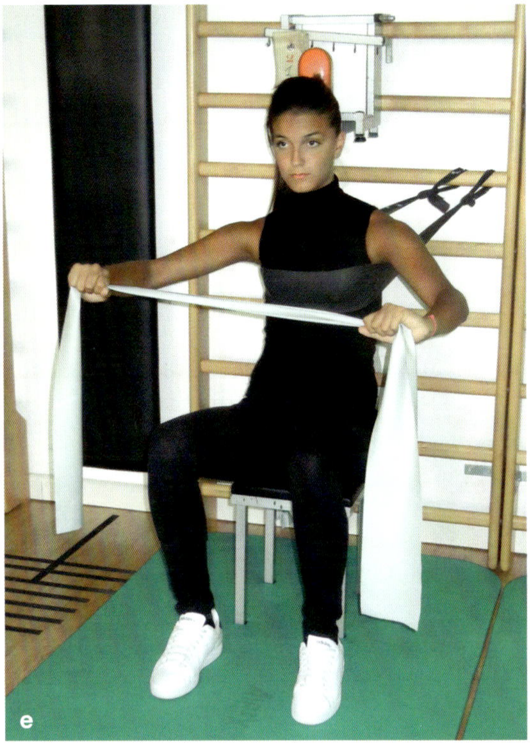

Variant - This exercise may be executed with a variant that makes it more difficult. Sitting on the Swiss ball helps the correction of the compensatory curve. The use of a more resistant elastic band (light grey color) on the chest makes the exercise more difficult. We remind the reader that the choice of elastic bands (which differ in color and resistance) concerns the therapist, who values their appropriateness in relation to the patient's situation.

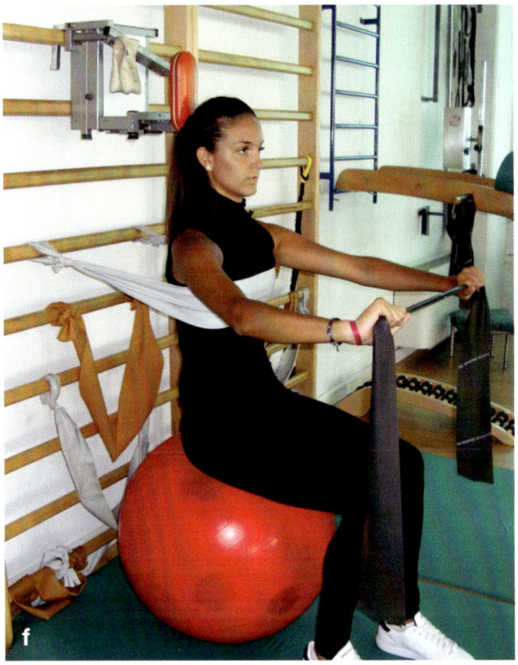

EXERCISE 5.20

Three-dimensional Corrective
This exercise is kyphotizing and involves three-dimensional self-correction.

Execution - Light self-stretching is induced in a seated position, with a fixed point on the Magri self-extender and with the elastic band wrapping around the back (**a**); three-dimensional correction is performed (kyphotization, lateralization, and derotation; **b**).

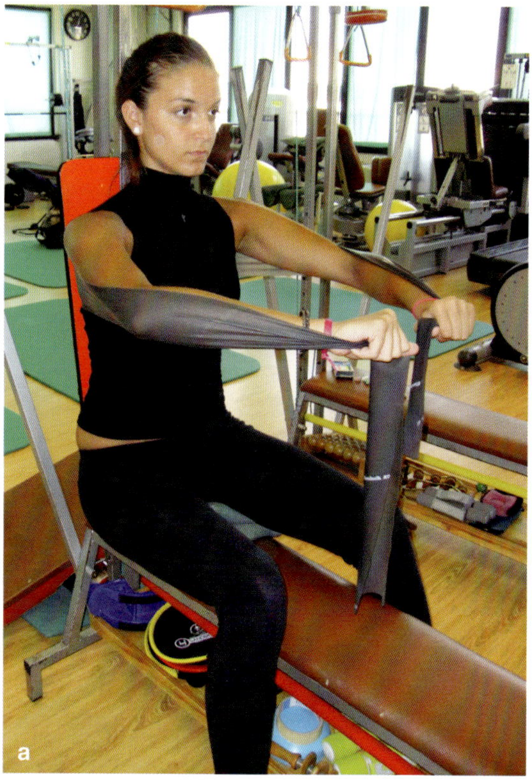

a

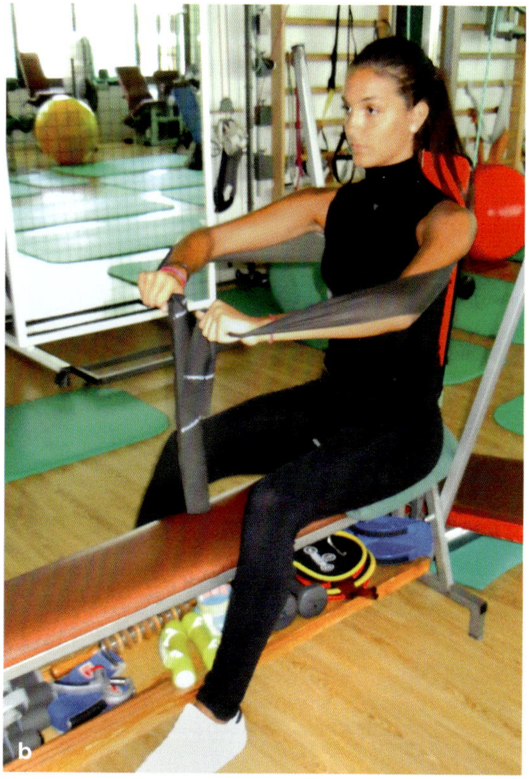

b

Magri self-extender - Conceived by Professor Magri and used in the seventies and eighties for self-stretching of the spine and self-correction. In this case, the device is applied to the Pivetta non-overturning bench. Additionally, positioned in front of the orthopedic mirror, the device facilitates self-correction.

EXERCISE 5.21

Muscular Strengthening
Abdominal muscular strengthening exercise with correction.

Execution - On the knees in front of the wall bars, the patient pulls the elastic band toward the body (at the knees), performing isometric contraction in the abdomen (core stability or lumbopelvic stabilization, **a**). Working during exhalation, a fulcrum is isometrically made with the hands; the patient pulls downward and seeks self-correction on the three planes of space: kyphotization, lateralization, and derotation (**b**).

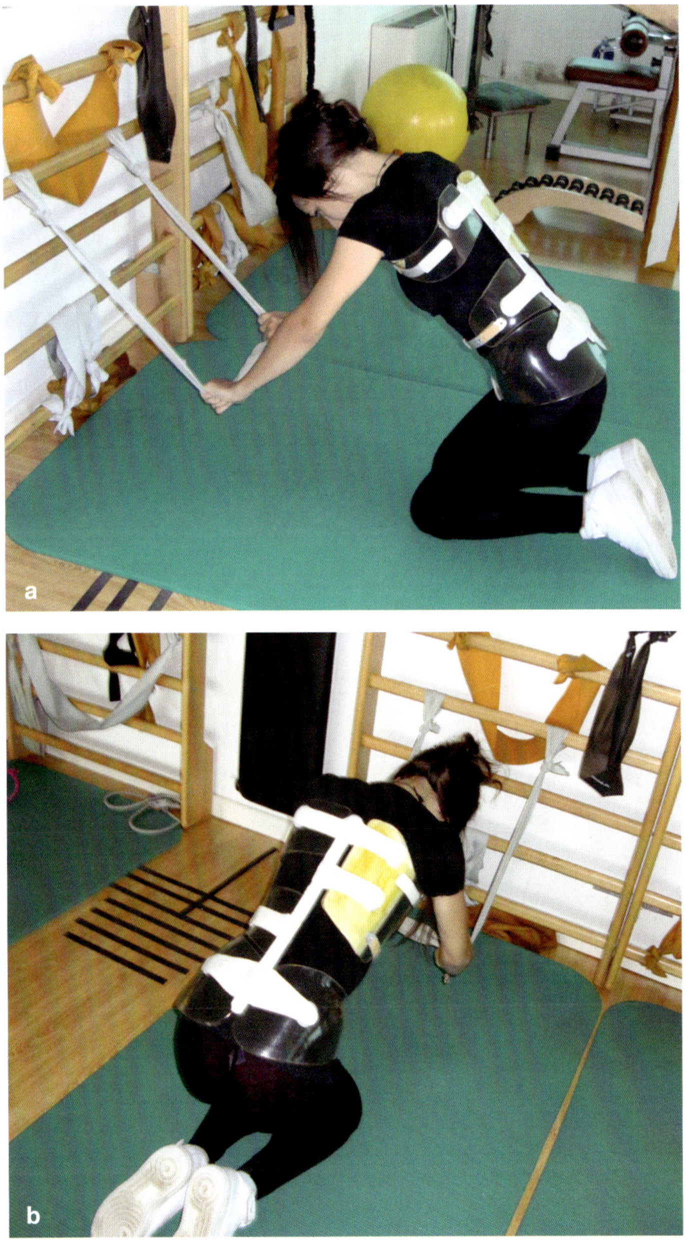

EXERCISE 5.22

Muscular Strengthening

Objective: strengthening of the muscles of the lower limbs.

Execution - An elastic band is tied in a ring of the appropriate size and then wrapped around the feet; the hands are on the hips. The patient alternately lifts the feet, keeping the elastic band in constant traction. The exercise is carried out with and without the corset.

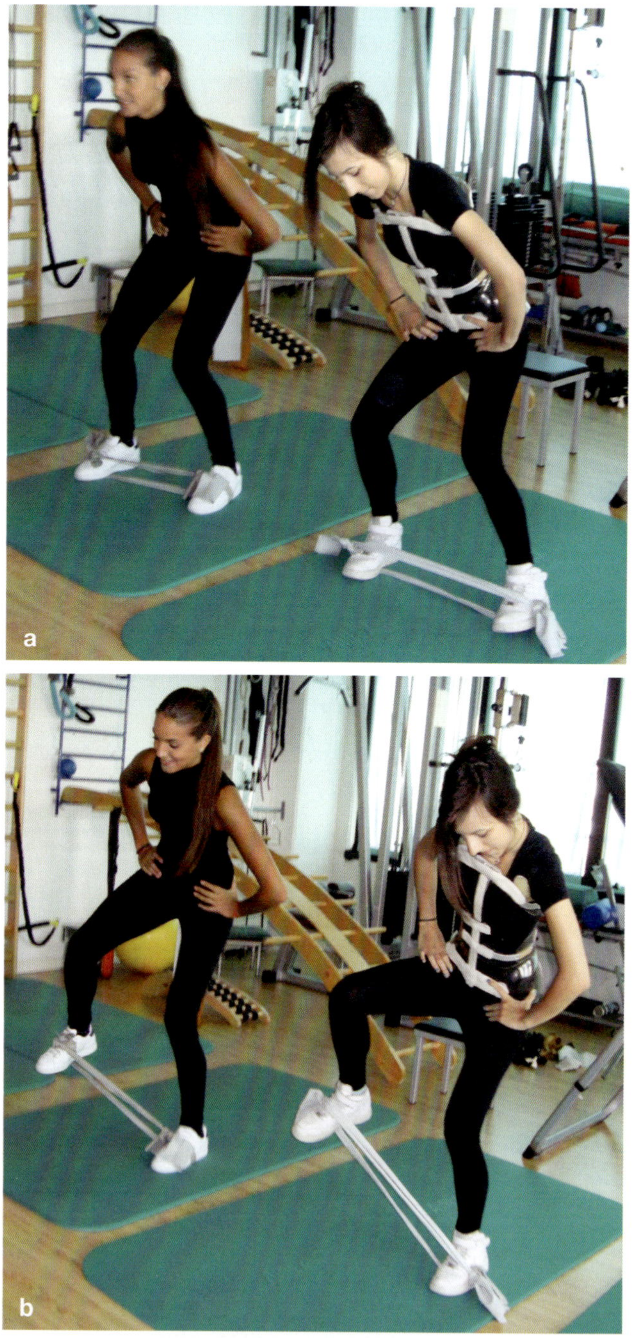

EXERCISE 5.23

Gaining Awareness and Strengthening

This is an exercise for gaining awareness of defects and muscular strengthening (paravertebral muscles).

Execution - In a seated position in front of the orthopedic mirror, with elastic placed over the head and held with the hands (which rest on the ground), the patient performs spinal stretching with control of the posture on the frontal plane. The cushion positioned under the gluteus is needed to compensate for any imbalances of the pelvis.
During exhalation, self-correction is performed via the three phases of kyphotization, lateralization, and derotation.

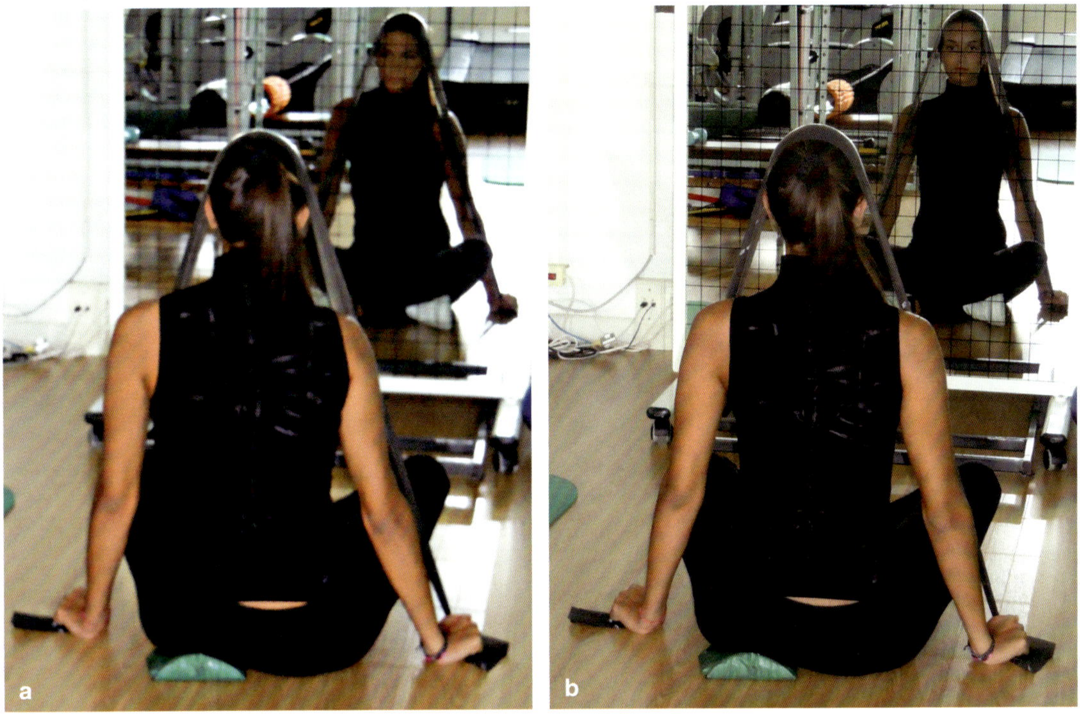

a, Starting position; **b**, three-dimensional correction: kyphotizing, lateralizing, and derotating.

EXERCISE 5.24

Corrective Destabilizing

Kinesiological view of the correction.

Execution - Seated in front of the mirror on a tilting board, the elastic is placed under the gluteus (**a**). The elbows are inserted into the elastic band, the trunk is brought slightly forward, and the patient performs three-dimensional correction (kyphotization, lateralization, and derotation) during prolonged exhalation (**b**, **c**). A cushion placed under the gluteus on one side may serve to reduce any lumbar compensation.

Beginning position (**a**); correction: posterior (**b**) and three-quarters view (**c**).

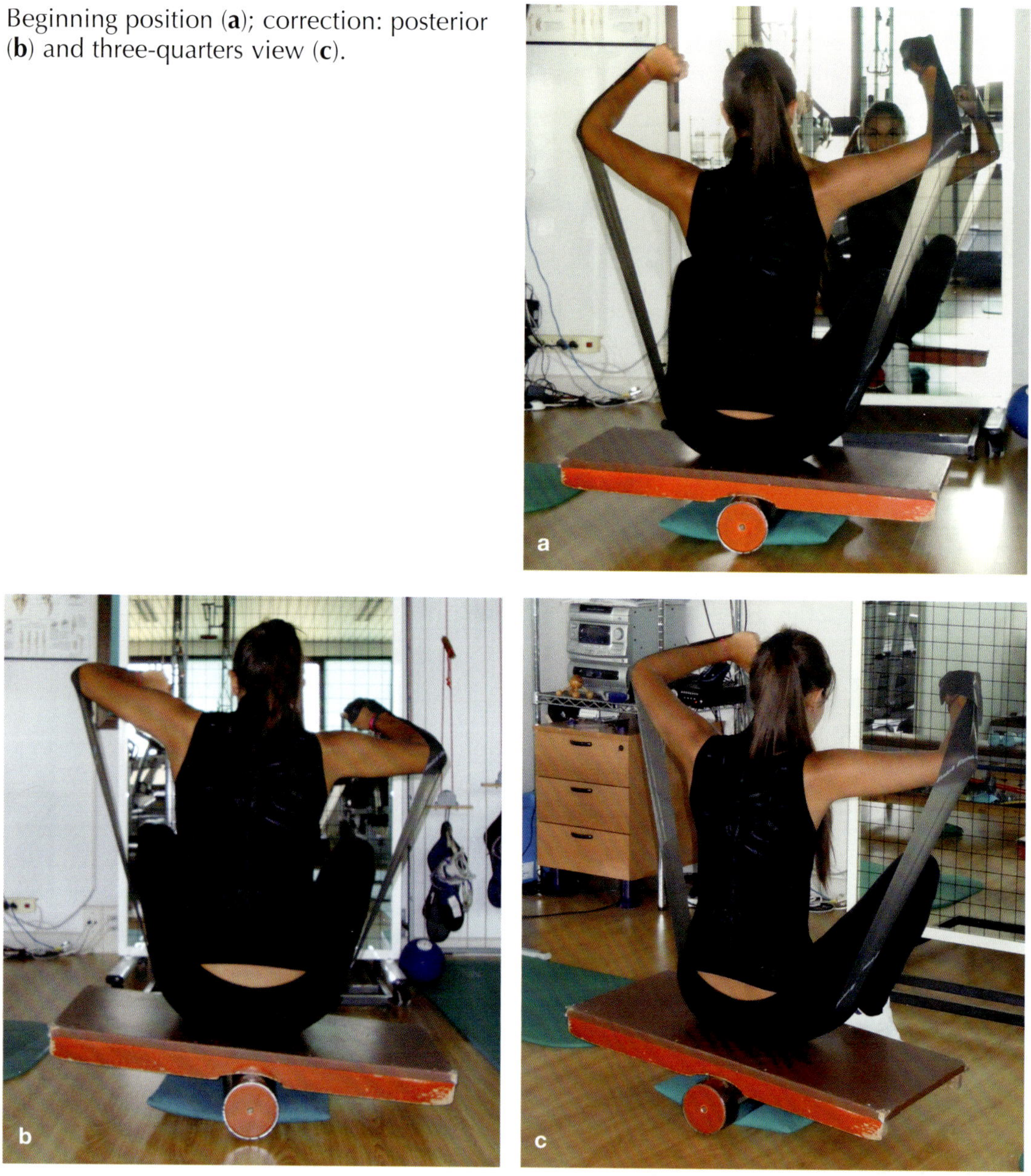

EXERCISE 5.25

Asymmetrical Corrective

The exercise is self-correcting of the dorsal hump.

Execution - With elastic bands wrapped around a high rung of the wall bars, the patient grips the elastic bands in an asymmetrical manner (with the higher hand opposite the dorsal hump in order to incentivize corrective movement, **a**, **b**). The body is in total load relief (**c**); the knees are flexed and rotated in the direction contralateral to the lumbar convexity (**d**).

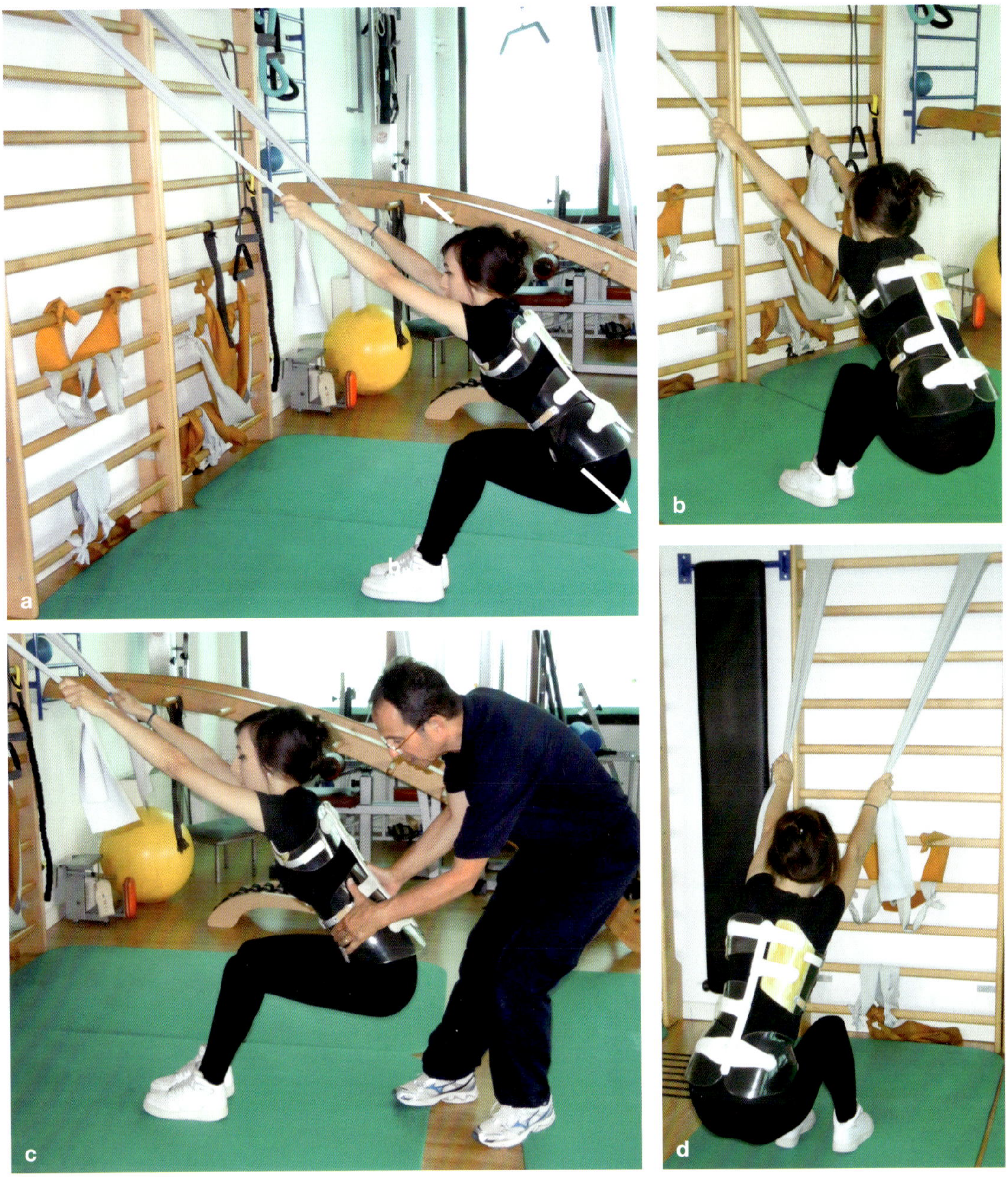

EXERCISE 5.26

Asymmetrical Corrective

The asymmetrical corrective exercise uses the *Ro-Plan Fly* device (a trademark of the Rovatti Plan®).

Execution - The patient uses the *Ro-Plan Fly* in order to attain vertebral unloading and relief of tension in the paravertebral muscles. Then, in full vertebral unloading, the patient performs correction on the three planes of space (kyphotization, lateralization, and derotation). The patient immediately feels a sensation of well-being at the dorsal-lumbar-sacral spine.

The exercise may be performed either with the corset (**a-d**) or without it (**e**, **f**).

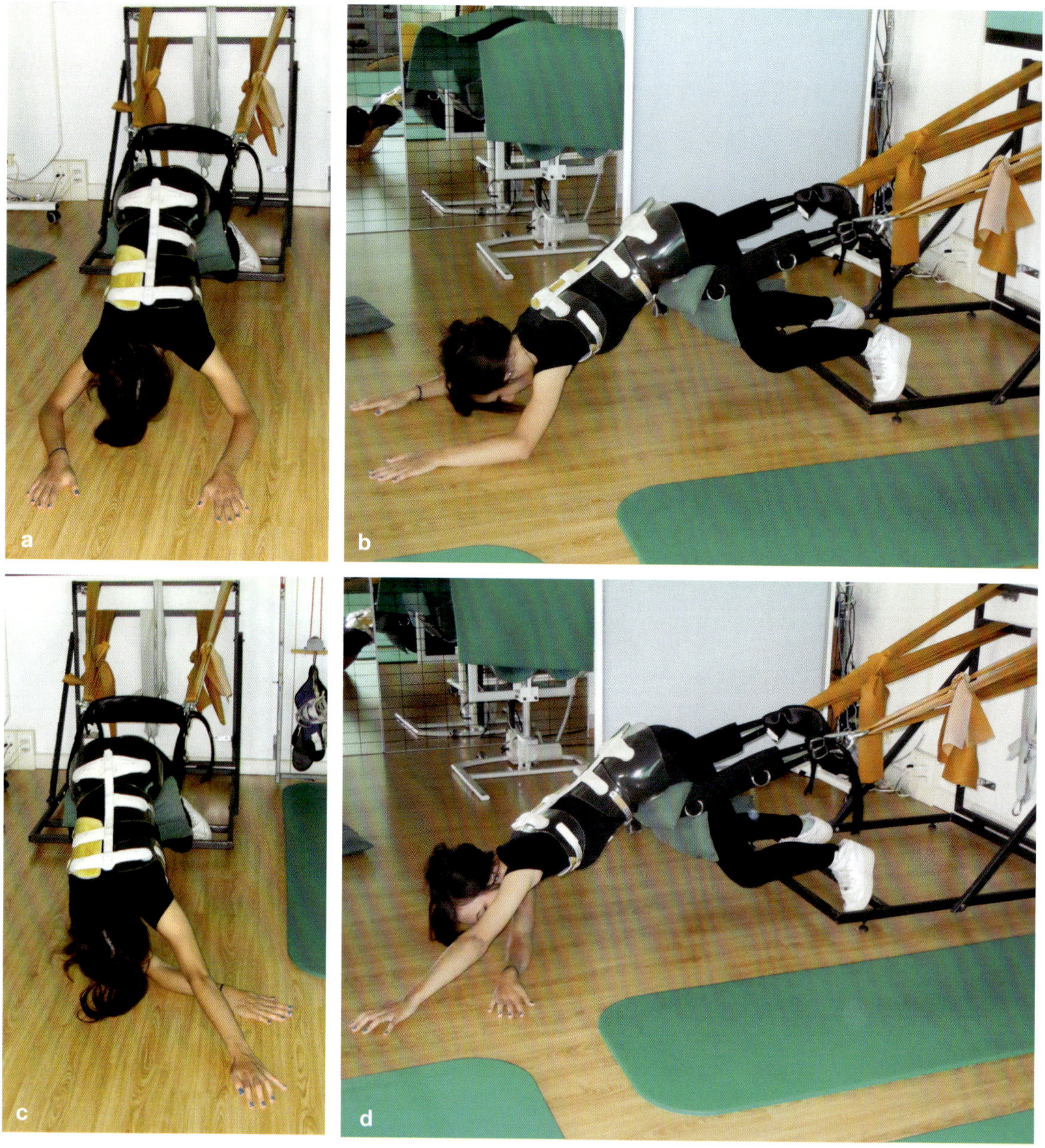

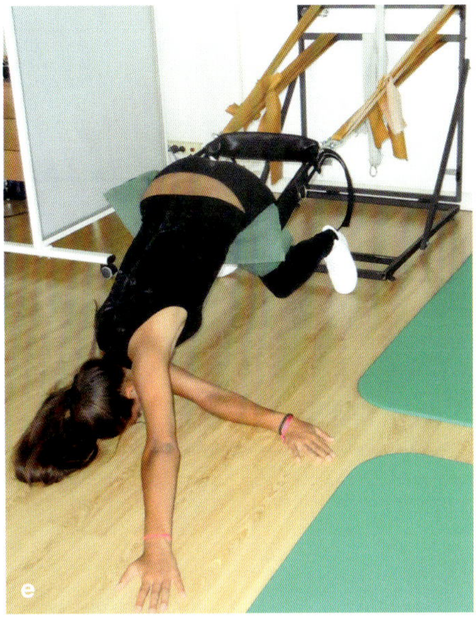

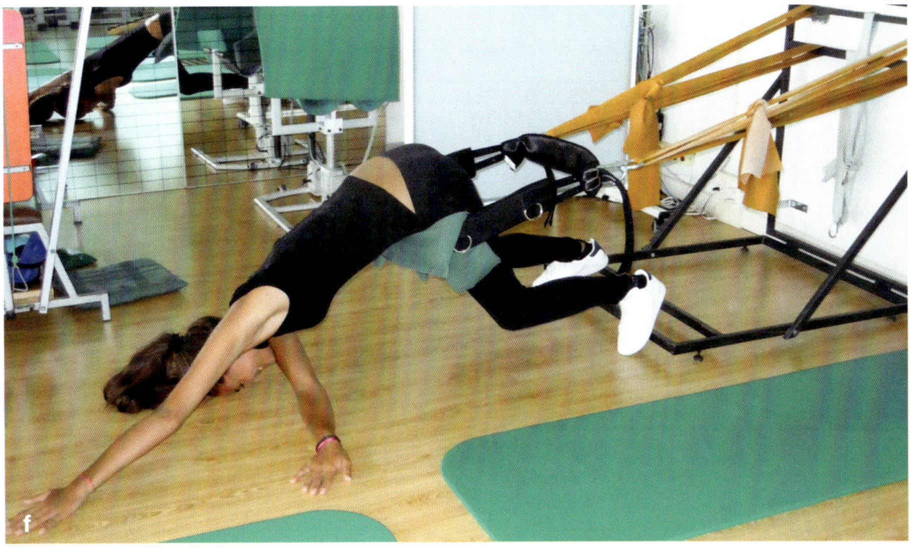

Ro-Plan Fly® - This instrument, conceived and patented as part of the Rovatti Plan®, facilitates the unloading of the vertebral column, which is useful for the treatment of vertebral pain. In this case, it is used as a dynamic stopping point for the pelvis and facilitates dorsal correction, also favoring the stoppage of the lumbar compensatory curve. Attentive evaluation of the weight/stature/physical strength of the patient is required to provide the necessary resistance and thus the elastic to be used. The device's usefulness is owed to the ability to modulate in extension the lumbar spine both in kyphosis and lordosis, with great and immediate benefits. It is indicated for active tractions. There are immediate benefits, for example, in cases of back strain (lumbar antalgic position).

EXERCISE 5.27

Asymmetrical Corrective

This is an asymmetrical self-correction exercise. The elastic band facilitates three-dimensional correction.

Execution - The patient's body is positioned on top of the table, with the left hand slightly forward than the right in order to favor correction with a traction. A cylindrical cushion is placed under the abdomen, the elastic band is positioned over the area to be treated (wrapping around the dorsal hump), and the elbows are placed inside of the band (**a**). Kyphotization, lateralization, and derotation are performed. Any lumbar compensation may be helped by lateralizing the legs to the left (for a right lumbar compensatory curve) in slight suspension, with the knees slightly flexed and the lumbar region relieved of tension.

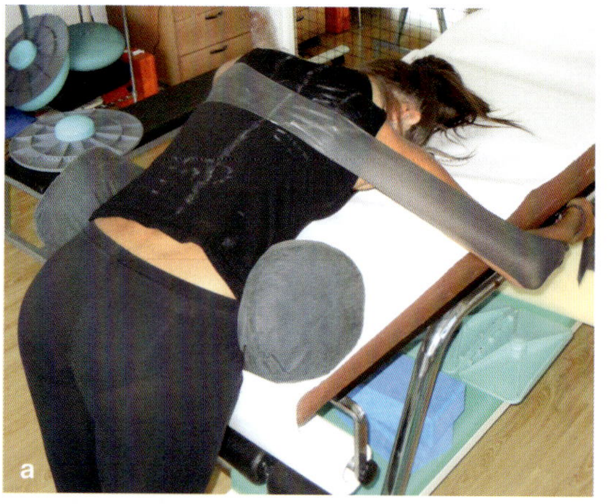
a

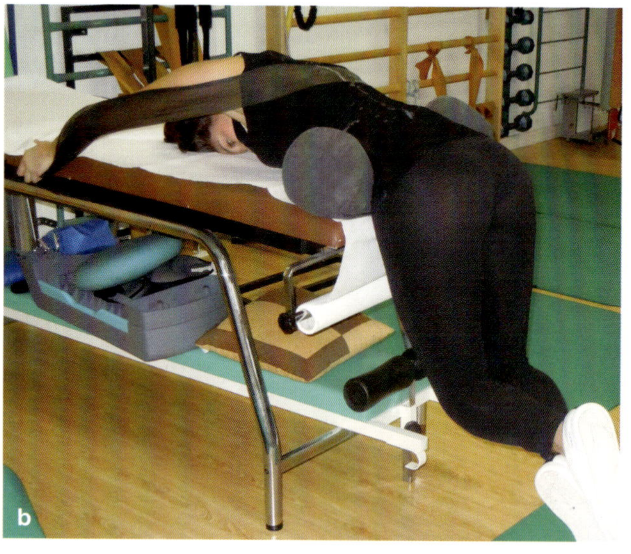
b

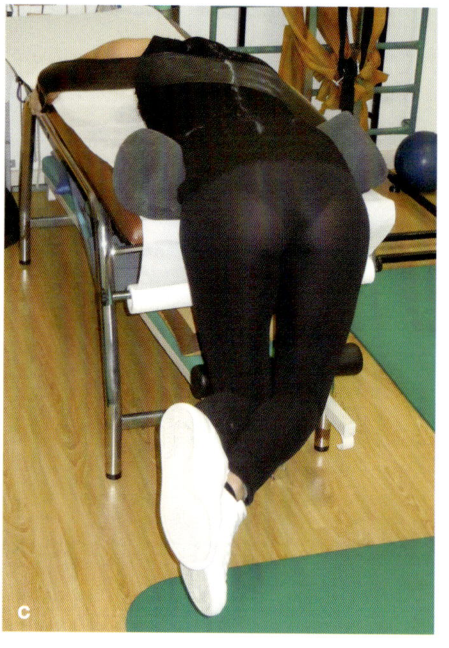
c

EXERCISE 5.28

Three-dimensional Corrective

This exercise is kyphotizing and induces three-dimensional correction of the dorsal curve and containment of secondary lumbar curves.

Execution - The patient sits with the right lower limb abducted (hurdler position) and the left resting on the wall bars to contain any lumbar compensatory curve. The elastic band, anchored to the wall bars, is wrapped around the scoliotic dorsal segment. The left arm is folded and placed over the opposite arm (**a**); with the trunk slightly inclined forward, three-dimensional correction is performed (**b**): kyphotization, lateralization, and derotation.

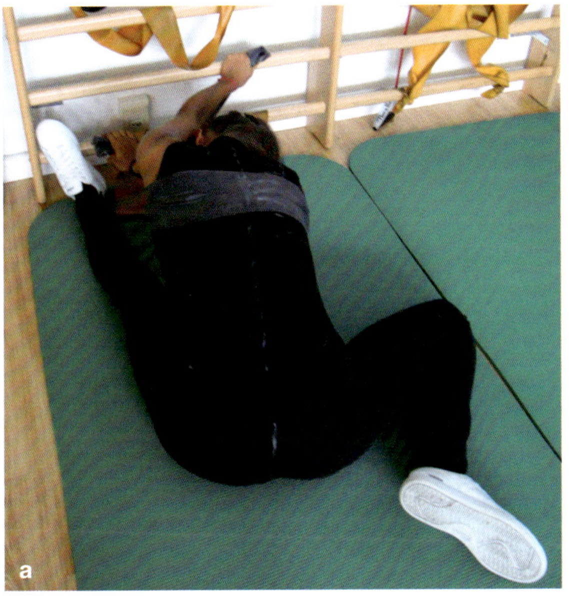
a

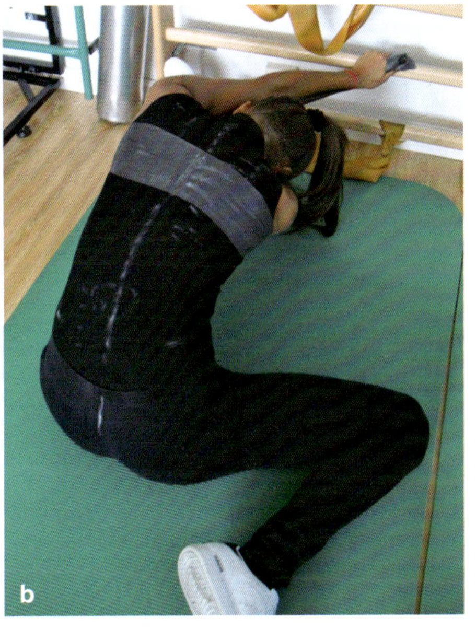
b

Variant - For purely right dorsal scoliosis cases, the patient is seated in front of the wall bars with the legs spread and the feet resting on the first rung (**c**).
The right arm remains on the second rung of the wall bars and provides a light push; the left arm is on the upper rung. Both ends of the elastic band, positioned over the dorsal hump, are held with the left hand, leaving the left elbow within the elastic band. The three-dimensional correction movement is performed with the right hand.
The containment of the opposing lumbar curve may be facilitated with the use of a spacer beneath the left gluteus and a small rhythmic gymnastics ball for decompressive effect from the side of the ribs, rotated anteriorly (left).

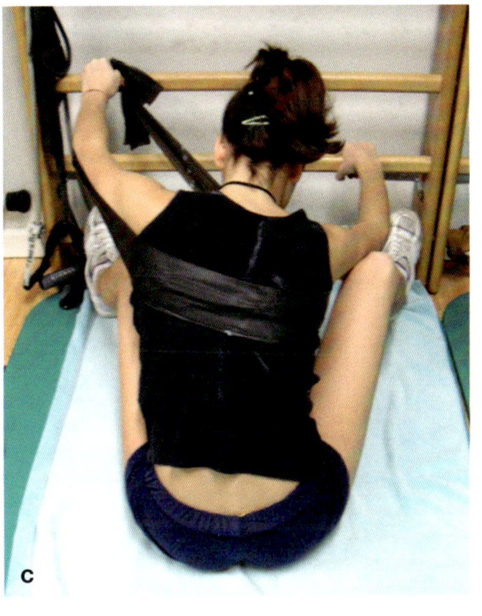
c

EXERCISE 5.29

Corrective

The objective of this exercise is the correction of the right dorsal hump.

Execution - The patient is seated on a Swiss ball in order to obtain the greatest degree of control of any lumbar compensatory curve. The two ends of the elastic band are anchored to the wall bars and to the dorsum of the right hand, and are brought into tension with the arms stretched in front of the patient. In this way, dorsal correction is facilitated during the execution of three-dimensional self-correction (**a**, **b**).

Variant - The same exercise is performed, but with retroposition of the right leg to additionally control any lumbar compensation (**c**).

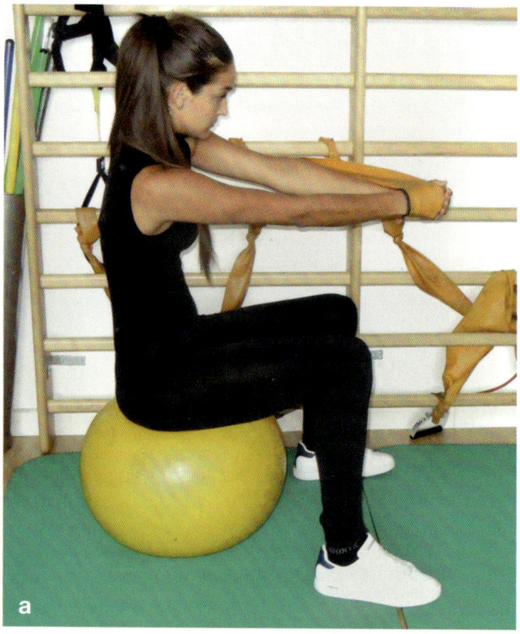

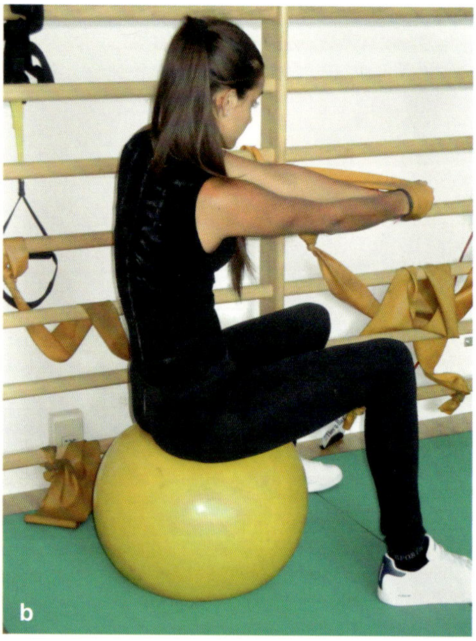

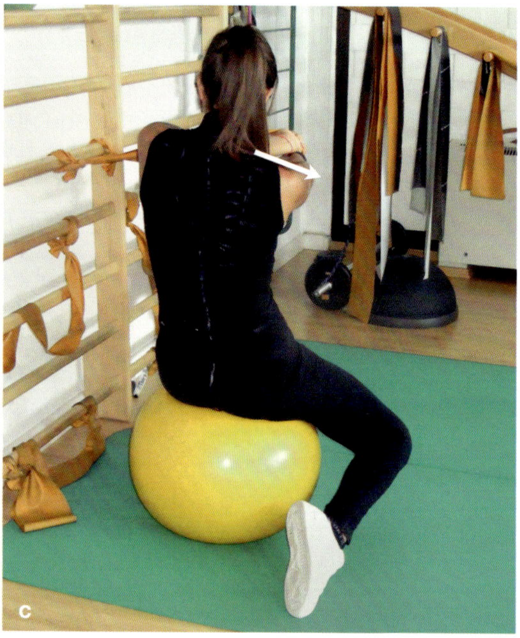

EXERCISE 5.30

"Niederhöffer"-type Corrective Exercise

Corrective exercise with corset for right dorsal hump.

Execution - The patient sits on a Swiss ball with the legs crossed, next to the wall bars: using a strong isometric contraction, the patient pulls toward the median axis of the body an elastic band of medium resistance that is anchored to the wall bars and hooked around the elbow of the left arm (**a**). The activation of the transverse muscles of the concavity of the curve causes these muscles to bring the vertebrae nearer the median line with corrective action. This exercise is to be performed during the exhalation phase via kyphotization, lateralization, and derotation. With proper execution, patients wearing the corset should perceive the reduction of the contact with the dorsal pelota.

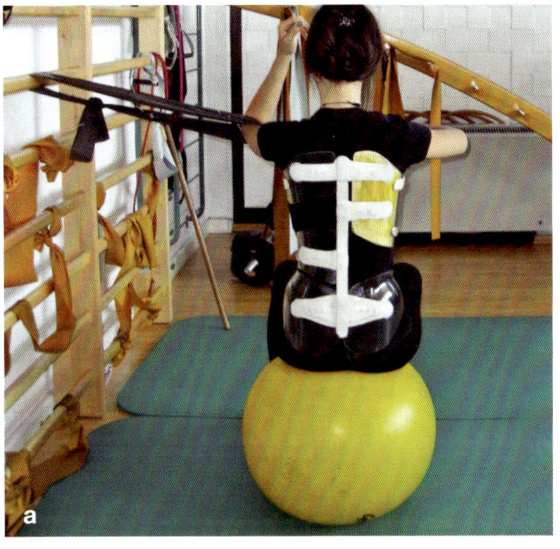
a

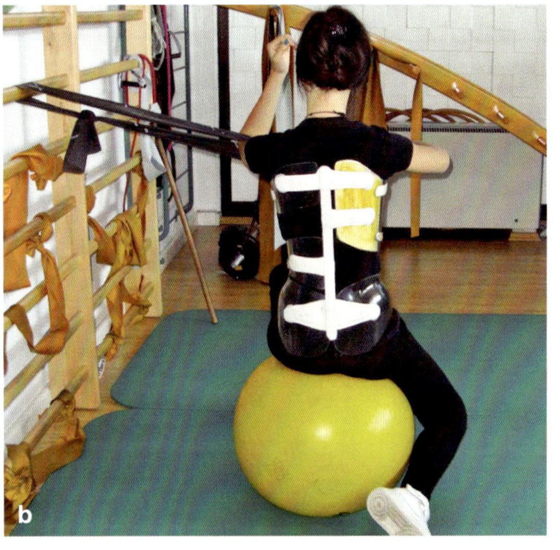
b

Variant - The same exercise is performed, but with retroposition of the right leg to further control any lumbar compensation (**b**, **c**).

Niederhöffer corrective techniques - The Niederhöffer method for the treatment of scoliosis introduces the concepts of resistance to external forces/traction and patient's active participation in a proprioceptive sense. The method makes use of the transverse muscles of the concavity of the scoliotic curve so that the contraction of these muscles brings the vertebrae nearer the median line with a corrective isometric action. The method was conceived in Germany at the beginning of the twentieth century by the neurologist von Niederhöffer, and spread through Italy in the first half of the 1970s.

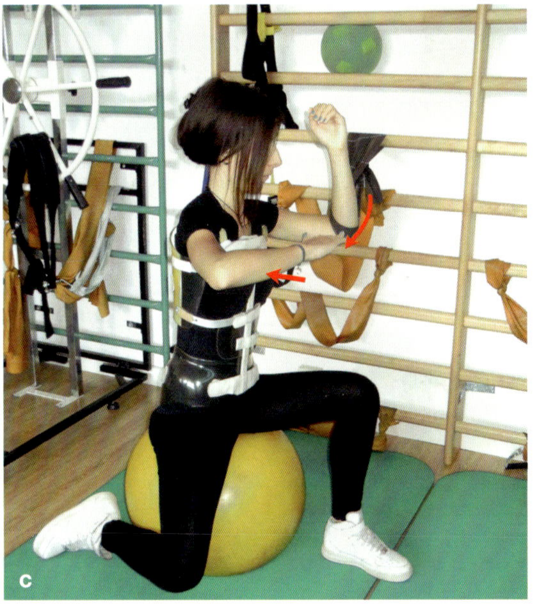
c

Group B

Group C

EXERCISE 5.31

"Niederhöffer"-type Corrective Exercise

Performed without a corset, "Niederhöffer"-type exercises are corrective for dorsal humps.

Execution - The elastic band, fixed to the wall bars, is brought into tension by placing it over the hump in such a way as to favor the direction of the correction.
The patient, seated on a Swiss ball, pulls toward the body with the arm gripping the rung of the wall bars in order to obtain a derotating contraction of the column. The right arm favors kyphotization. This exercise is entirely performed during slow and prolonged exhalation.

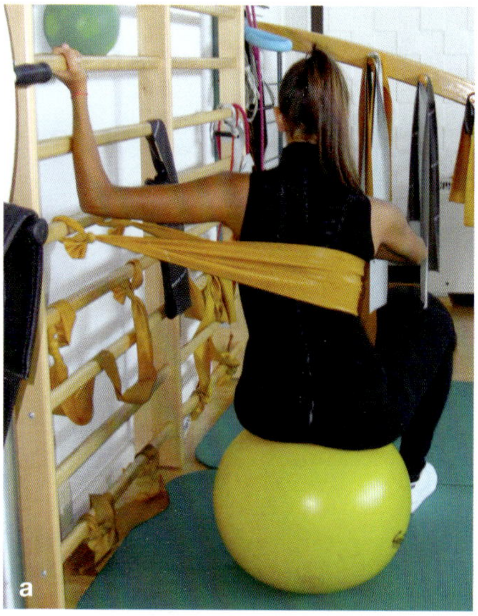

Variant - The same exercise is performed, but with retroposition of the right leg allowing any lumbar compensation to be further controlled (**b**, **c**).

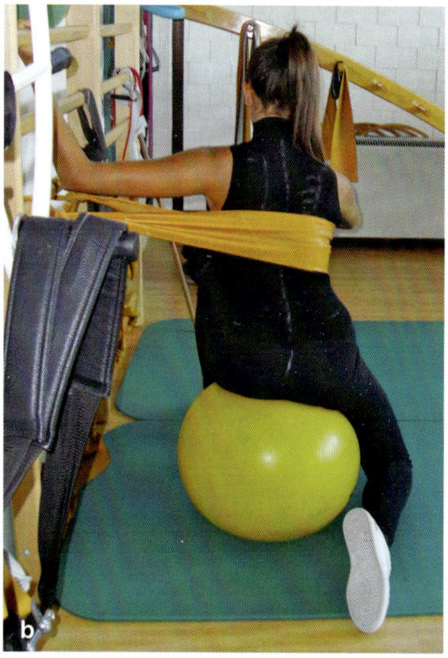

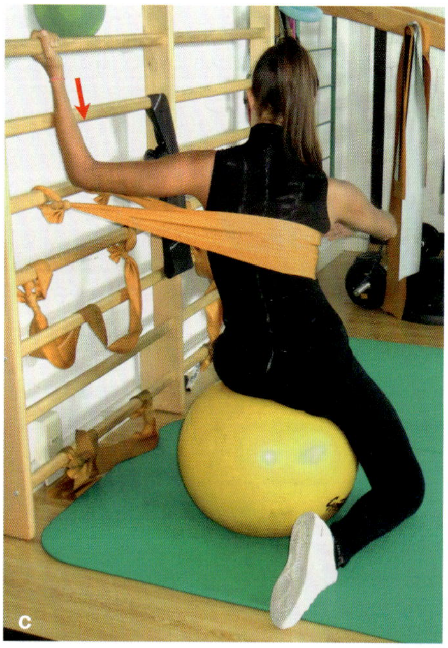

EXERCISE 5.32

Corrective

The exercise is kyphotizing and corrective, with the aim of three-dimensional correction of the curve.

Execution - With the patient positioned laterally to the wall bars sitting on a Swiss ball, the two ends of the elastic band hooked around the rung of the wall bars, the band passing around the trunk and wrapping the area of the dorsal hump. A medicine ball is held in the hands (arms forward). Kyphotization is promoted by two-handed pressure on the medicine ball (**a**). The elastic band, placed under strong tension, facilitates correction (**b**).

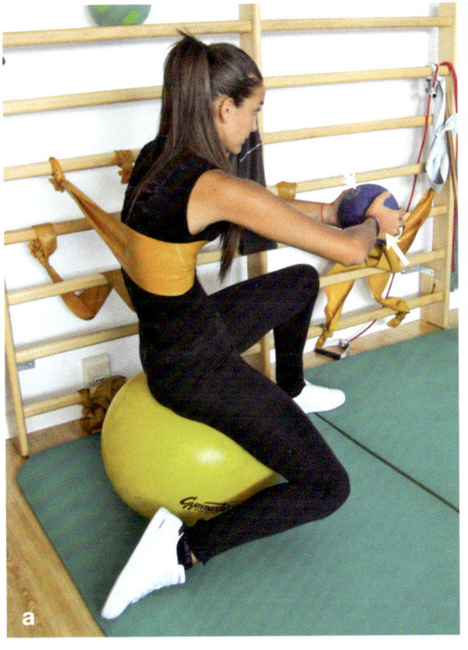
a

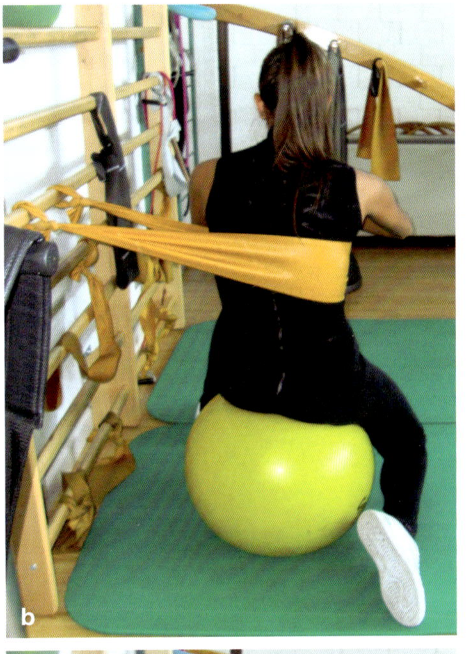
b

Variant - The exercise is similar to the preceding one, but the patient is seated on a stool and compensates the lumbar curve with a cushion under the left gluteus (**c**).

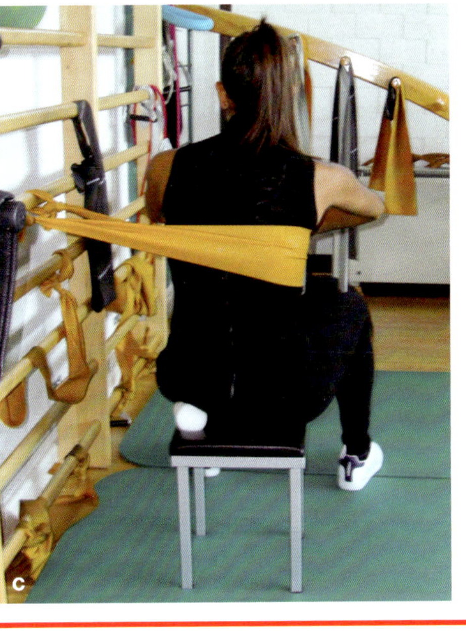
c

Group B

Group C

EXERCISE 5.33

Corrective
This exercise is corrective on the three dimensional planes, and particularly seeks dorsal correction and containment of the lumbar curve.

Execution - With the patient seated on a Swiss ball in front of the wall bars in order to have optimal lumbar control, the left foot rests upon the rung while the right leg is in retroposition. The elastic band wraps around the dorsal hump and is anchored (both ends) with the left hand on the rung of the wall bars at the height of the head, in order to obtain a tension-traction force that encourages three-dimensional correction. The exercise is performed during exhalation with the trunk slightly forward. The following are done in order: kyphotization, lateralization, and derotation (**a**, **b**).

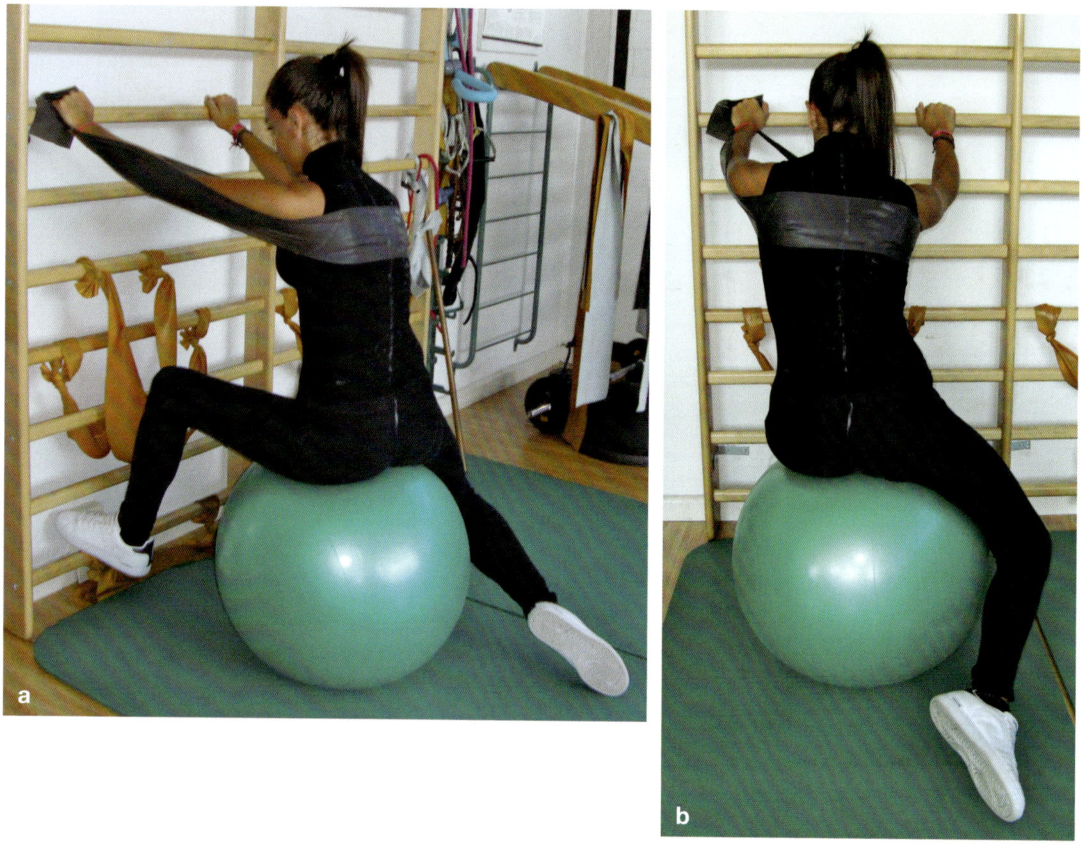

EXERCISE 5.34

Corrective

The exercise is corrective and kyphotizing with the gaining of consciousness of defects and proprioceptive sensations. It provides control of the pelvis in neutral position.

Execution - This exercise may only be carried out by an experienced patient due to its complexity. The elastic band, held in the hands, must wrap around the back of the Swiss ball, on which the patient lies as well. The elbows stay within the band. The legs are bent at around 90 degrees, with the feet resting on the rung of the wall bars (**a**, **b**). In order to reach the starting position (**a**), the patient must slide their back along the surface of the ball. With the dorsal support on the Swiss ball providing a proprioceptive stimulus, the patient performs the corrective adjustments using the upper limbs as a point of reference for the refinement of the correction (**b**). The support of the feet on a higher level of the wall bars may be used to control any lumbar compensatory curve (**c**).

Variant - The elastic band may also be placed directly under the back (**d**); in this image, the patient must still "slide" on the ball with the back in order to reach the starting position.

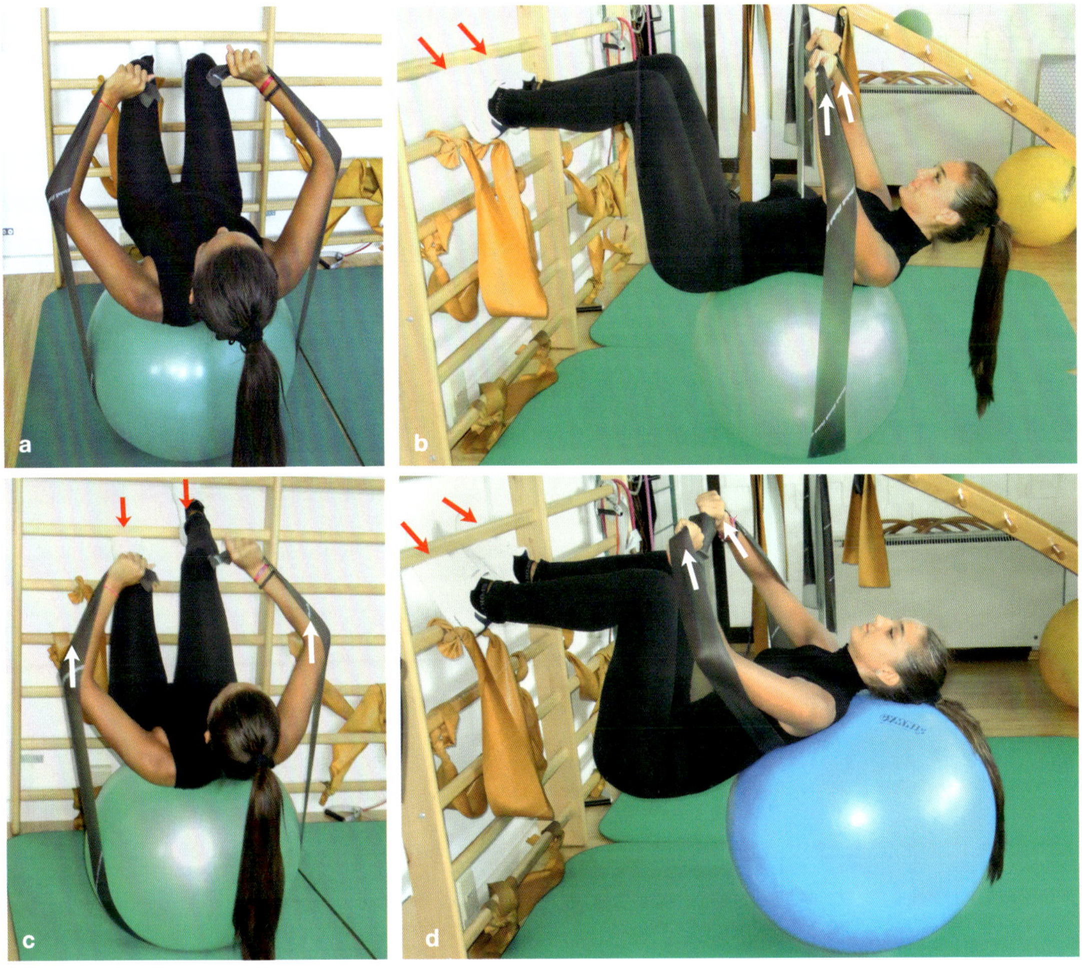

Group B

Group C

EXERCISE 5.35

Corrective

This exercise allows for three-dimensional correction of the primary dorsal curve and the containment of the lumbar counter-curve.

Execution - Seated on the "Pivetta non-overturning bench", the patient grasps the two ends of the elastic band (which wraps around the area of the dorsal hump) with the left hand (**a**). The hand pulls in the direction of the correction via a derotatory movement of the left elbow (note: the elastic wraps around the elbow), the trunk is flexed forwards, and the right hand orients the corrective direction, making a fixed point on the bench (**b**, **c**).

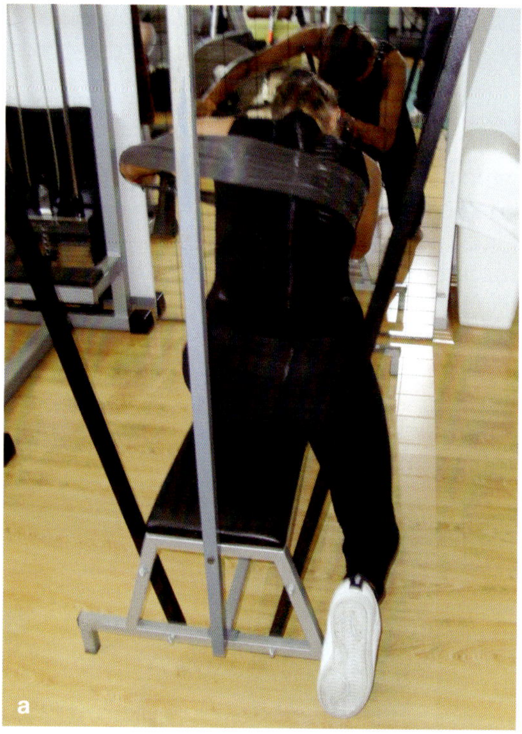

a

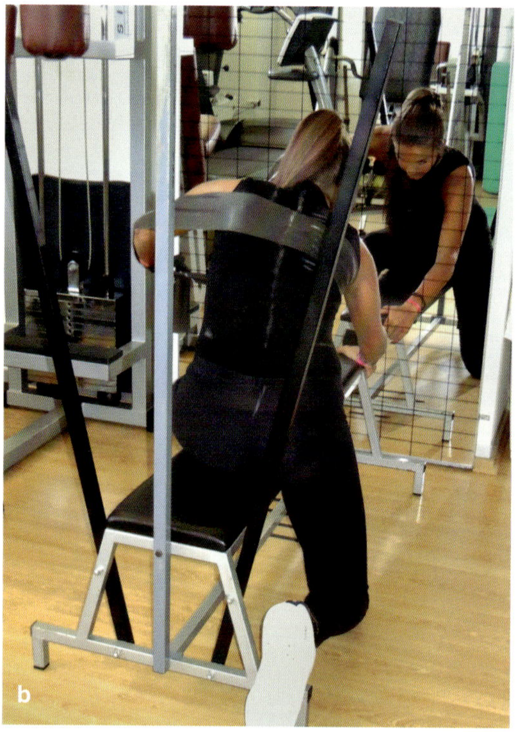

b

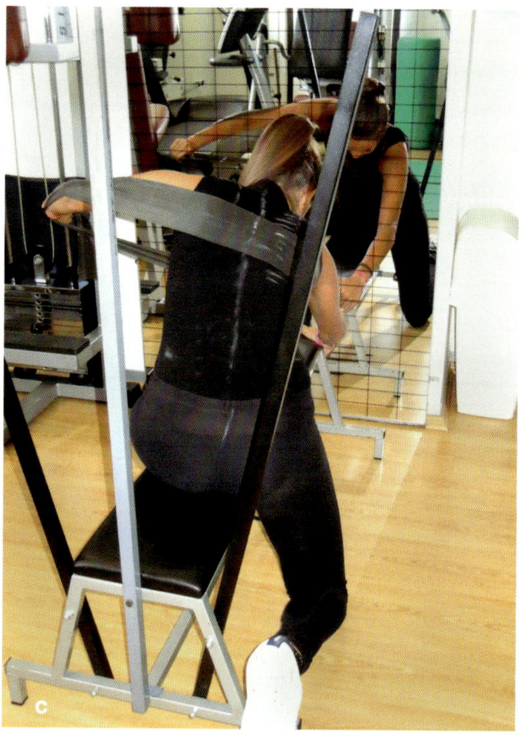

c

Variant - The left hand grips both ends of the elastic band in order to obtain a greater force effect. In this case, the right hand pulls in the direction opposite that of the left hand, supporting the three-dimensional correction movement. For thoracic scoliosis, the last ribs are rotated clockwise and are "horizontalized" (**d**). A medicine (or rhythmic gymnastics) ball placed between the left thigh and the abdomen contains any worsening of the ribs.

d, Preparation of the exercise;
e, correction, lateral view;
f, correction, posterior frontal view.

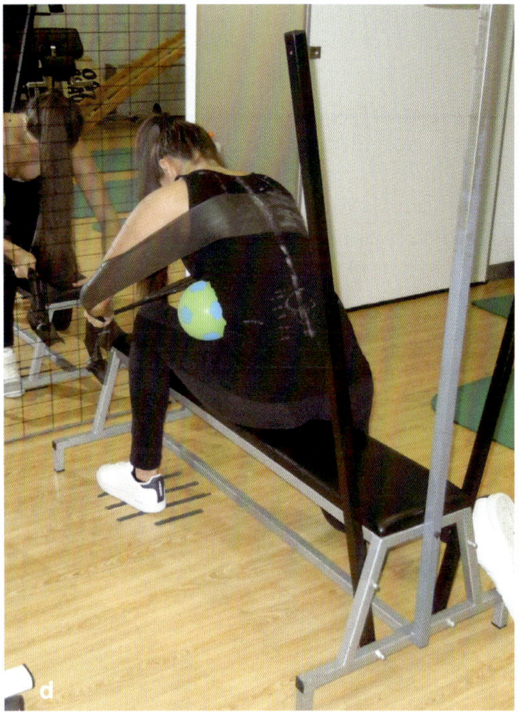

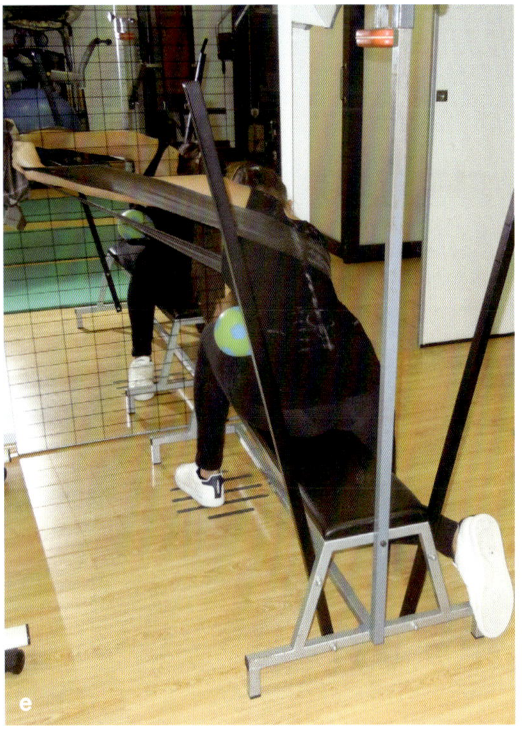

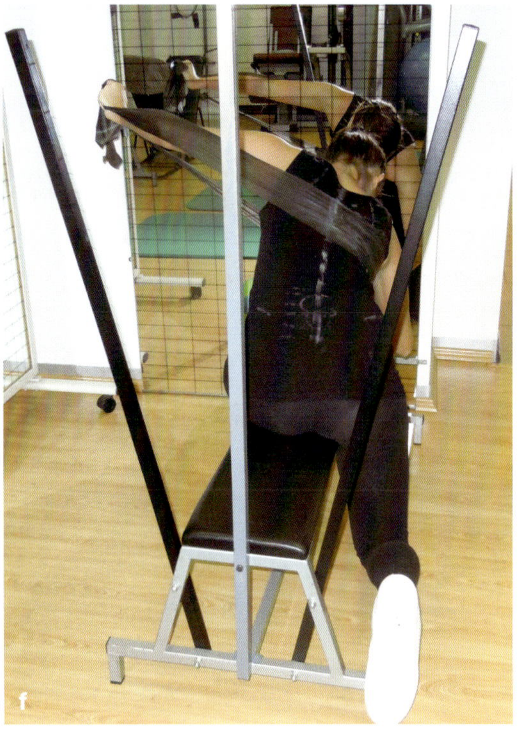

EXERCISE 5.36

Corrective and Strengthening

The execution of this exercise leads to the correction and activation of the paravertebral muscles.

Execution - The elastic band is positioned under the sole of the left foot, with the leg in lunge position and the trunk inclined forward; the right leg is aligned with the right half of the back; the elbows are wrapped around, respectively, by the two ends of elastic held with the two hands. The patient produces slight kyphotization of the back during exhalation (**a**) and subsequent lateralization (**b**) and derotation (**c**). This exercise may be performed with and without the corset (**d**, **e**).

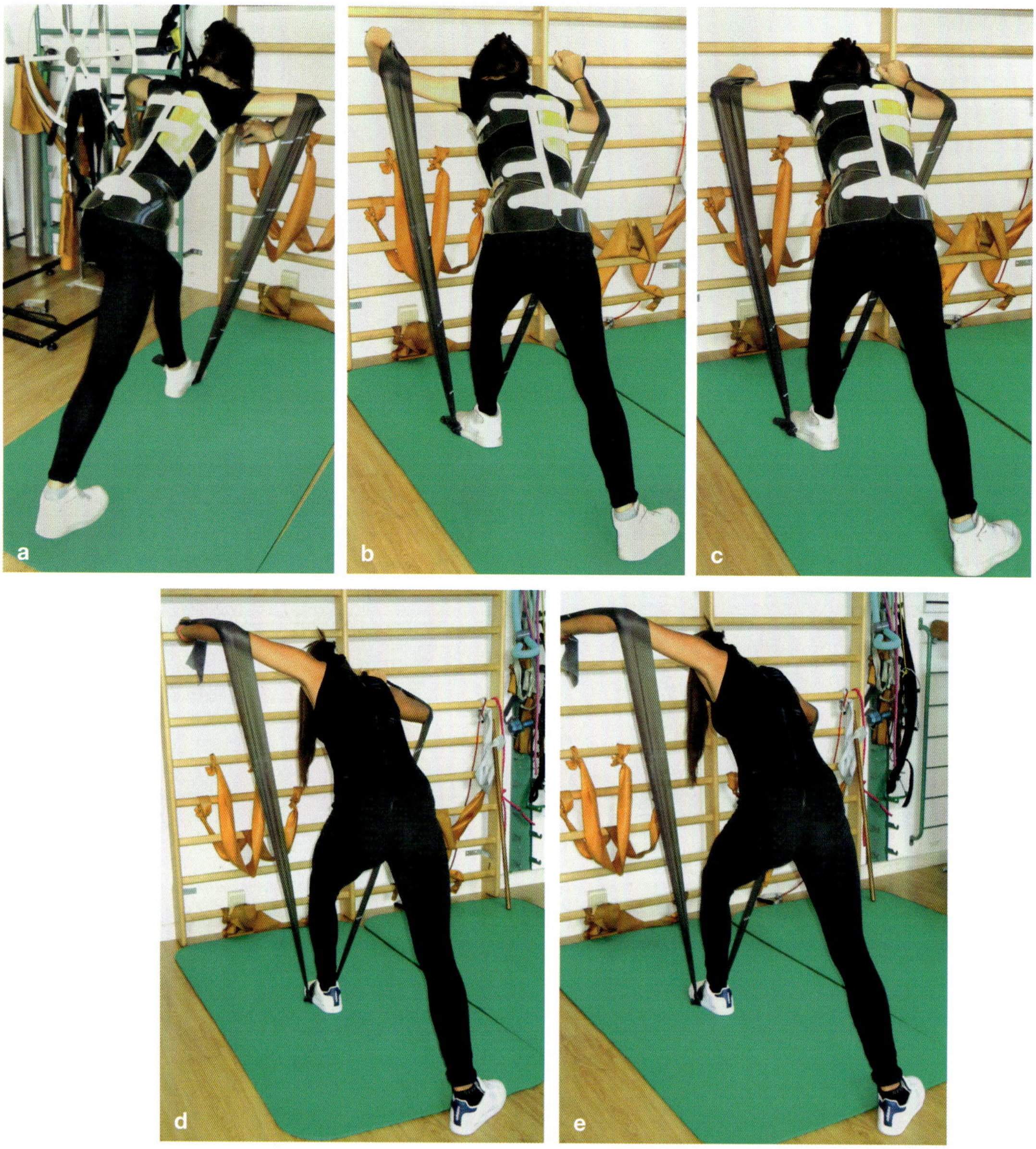

EXERCISE 5.37

Cross-country Skiing

The objective of this exercise is aerobic strengthening, general muscular strengthening, and monitoring of sensations while wearing the corset.

Execution - With elastic bands under the feet, perform rhythmic bending and extension of the lower limbs with alternating coordination of the upper limbs (simulation of the technical movement of cross-country skiing).

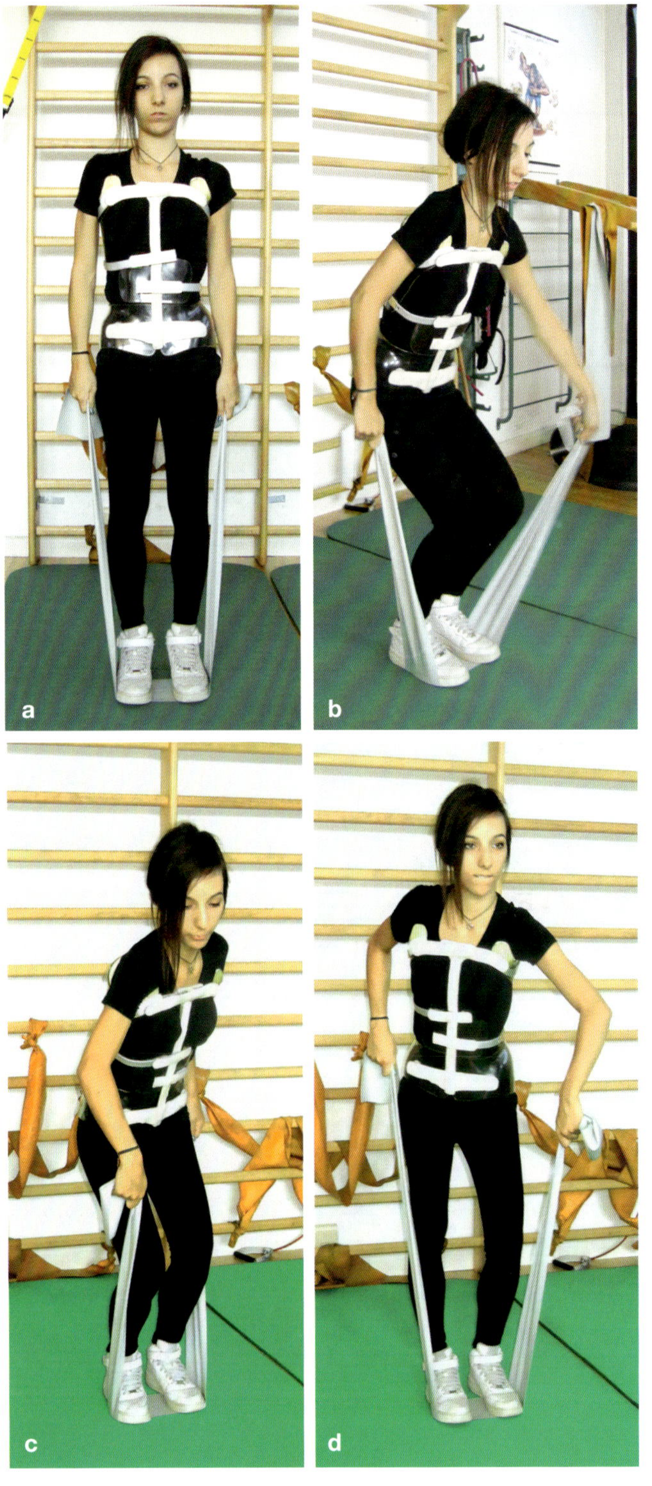

Group B

Group C

EXERCISE 5.38

Corrective

The objective of this exercise is the self-correction of the dorsal hump with compensation of the lumbar counter-curve.

Execution - With the patient in supine position, head towards the wall bars, a first elastic band, hooked around the fourth highest rung of the wall bars, is placed below the nape of the neck in order to relax the muscles; a second band is placed behind the heels (with the lower limbs bent by 90 degrees) in order to relieve tension in the posterior chain; then the feet are rotated to the right, and any compensatory curve is corrected. A third elastic band is grasped with the left hand (this band is hooked around a rung at the same height as the first band) in order to facilitate the correction of the right dorsal hump. The four pictures are frontal views of the same exercise, for its improved interpretation.

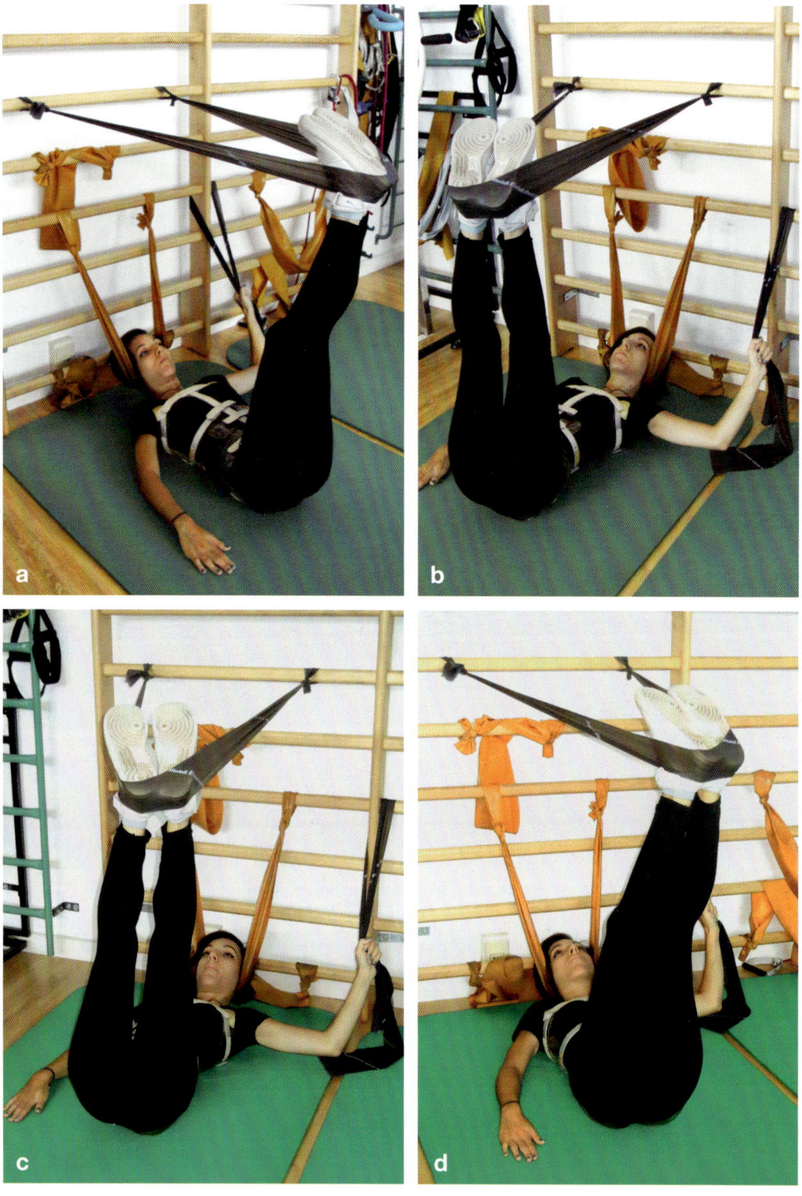

EXERCISE 5.39

Non-compensated Overall Stretching

This exercise is three-dimensional corrective, performed in a position of non-compensated stretching. This exercise may be performed both with and without the corset.

Execution - With the patient in supine position, head toward the wall bars, and lower limbs bent at 90 degrees, a first elastic band is hooked around the fourth rung of the wall bars and positioned below the nape of the neck in order to relax the muscles; a second band is placed behind the heels (the distance and tension of the elastic varies based on the patient's degree of preparation; **a**). With a third elastic band hooked around the fifth rung and grasped with both hands, it is possible to perform three-dimensional correction in a state of non-compensation (in sequence: kyphotization, lateralization, and then derotation; **b**).

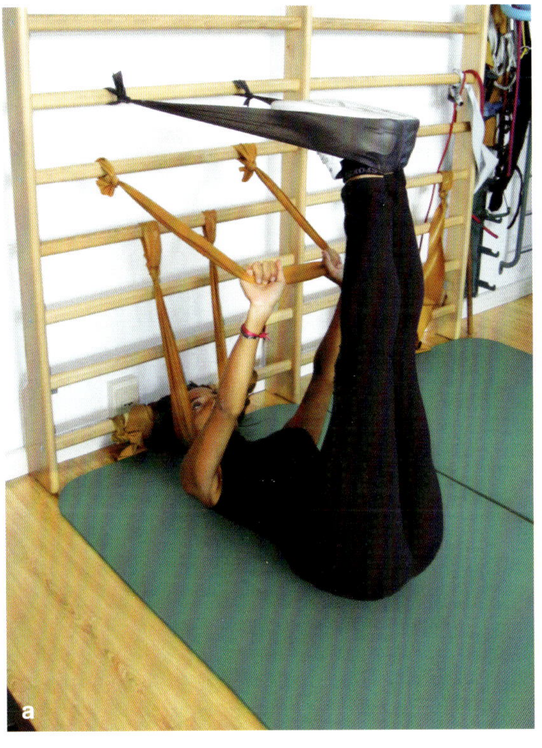
a

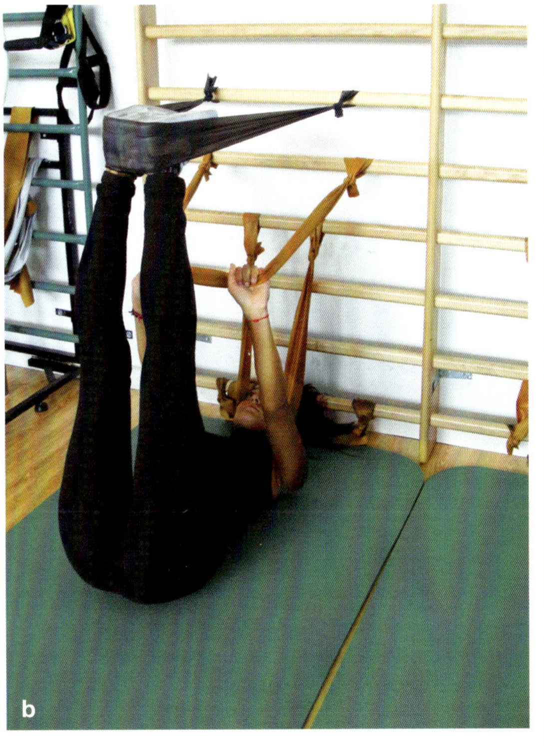
b

EXERCISE 5.40

Corrective

The objective of this exercise is the correction of the dorsal and lumbar curves. This exercise may be performed both without (**a**) and with (**b**) the corset.

Execution - The patient is in supine position, feet toward the wall bars. The right lower limb pulls on an elastic anchored to the wall bars and to the knee in order to obtain activation of the psoas muscle. The left hand uses a baton as a fixed point to facilitate dorsal movement during the attempt at correction of the curves (kyphotization, lateralization, and derotation).

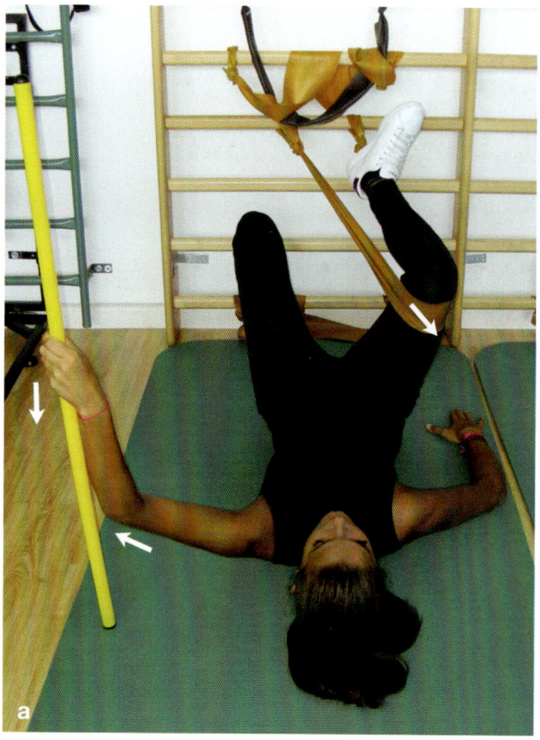

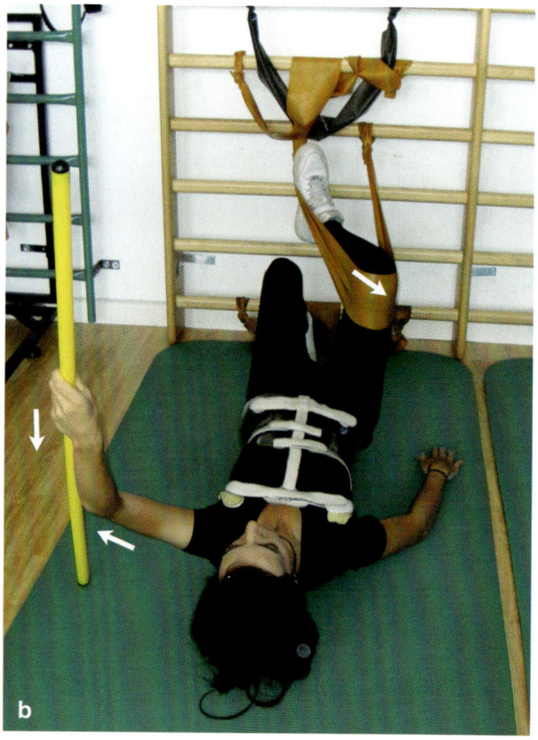

EXERCISE 5.41

Corrective

This exercise is performed for lumbar correction (right psoas muscle) and dorsal kyphotization with correction. The exercise is carried out with and without the corset. This exercise strongly stimulates trophism of the abdominal muscles as well.

Execution - The patient is in the supine position in front of the wall bars; a weight is added to the right ankle in order to stimulate the right psoas muscle. The patient kyphotizes and pulls with the arm holding the elastic band fixed to the wall bars above the head, seeking correction. The elastic band is used as a fixed point for correction, and in the meantime the patient kyphotizes, lateralizes, and derotates. The contact of the posterior part of the trunk with the ground facilitates perception, even minimal, of the correction. The right leg lifted beyond 60 degrees and slightly abducted facilitates, via the psoas muscle, the non-compensation of the secondary lumbar curve.

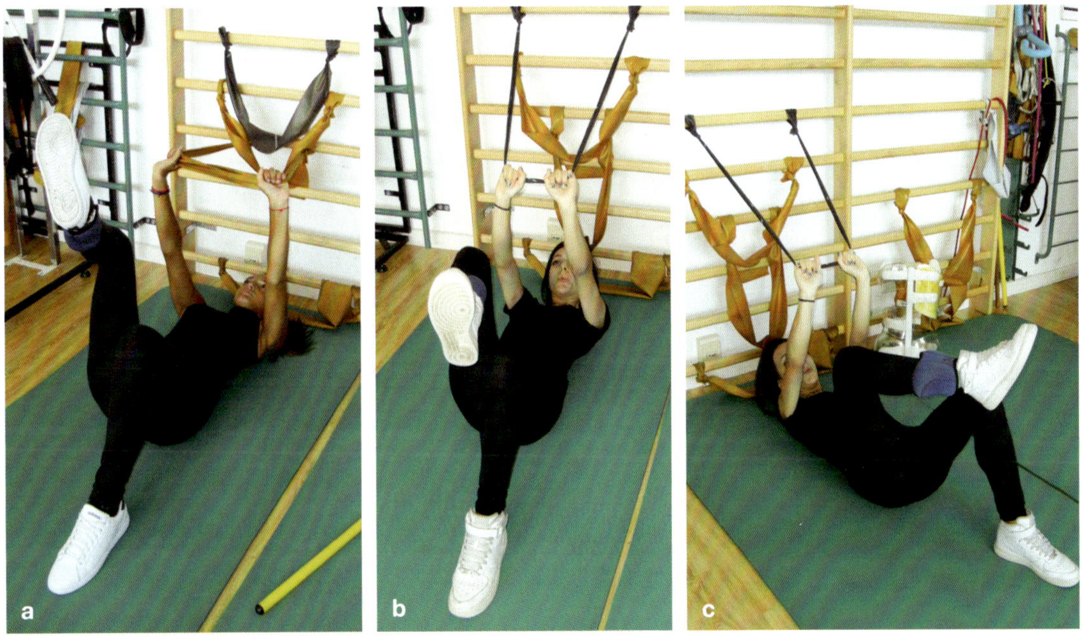

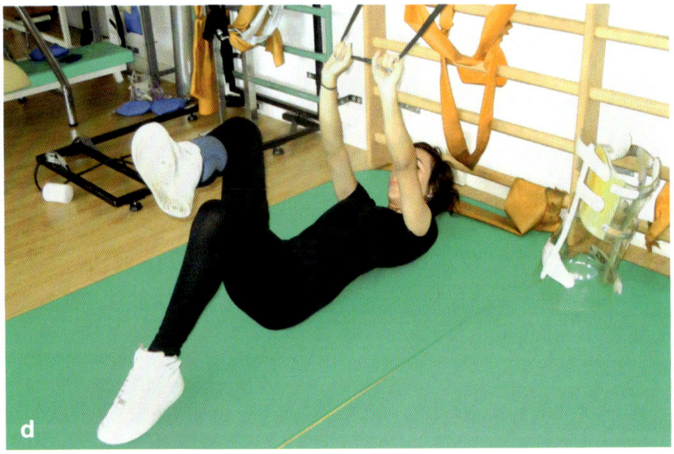

The elastic bands are differentiated by color/intensity and height of attachment at the therapist's discretion. In case **a**, the elastic band is more resistant, but is attached at a lower level.

Group B

Group C

EXERCISE 5.42

Corrective

Exercise for three-dimensional self-correction of the scoliotic curve.

Execution - The patient is seated on a Swiss ball positioned in front of the wall bars (in order to sensitize the correction). The elastic band, anchored to the wall bars, is positioned over the chest; the patient moves the trunk forward seeking kyphotization, lateralization, and then derotation (i.e., three-dimensional correction of the scoliotic curve). The left hand aids in three-dimensional correction. The right hand is placed on the ball to aid the movement. The right leg, brought in the posterior direction, corrects any compensatory curve.

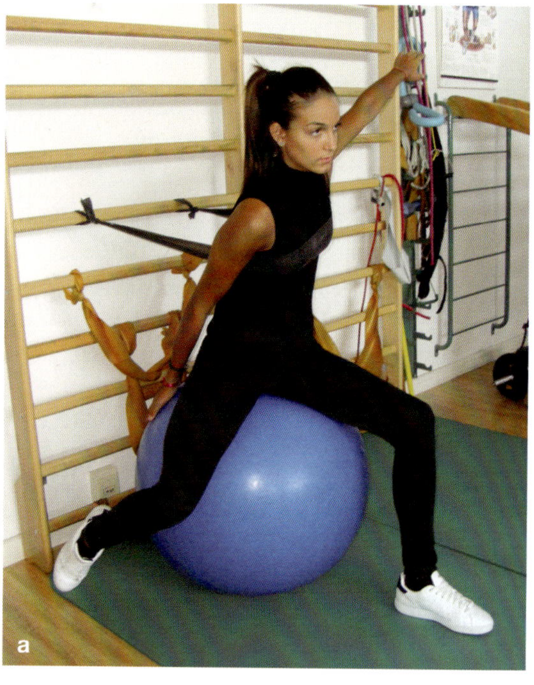

a

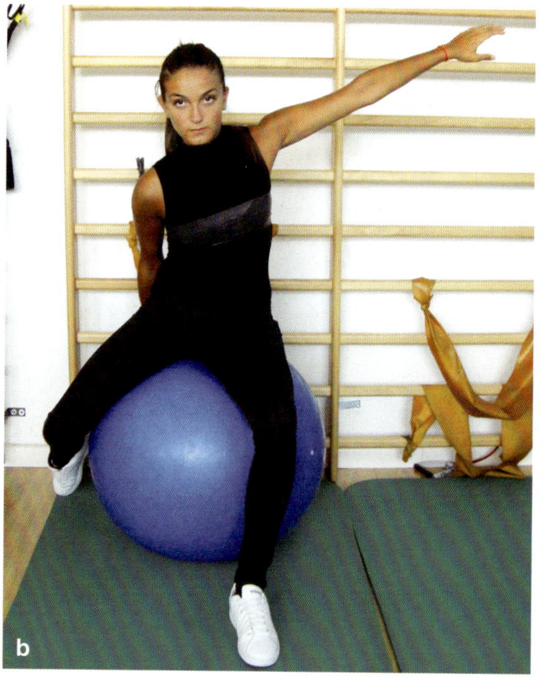

b

EXERCISE 5.43

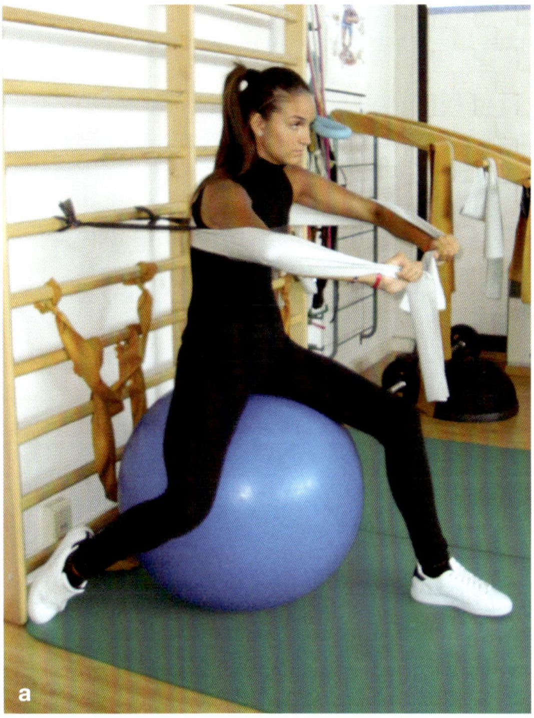

Corrective
Three-dimensional correction of the scoliotic curve.

Execution - With the patient seated on a Swiss ball in front of the wall bars, the first elastic band is hooked around a rung and positioned over the chest. A second elastic band is then wrapped around the back at the hump and the elbows; the trunk is slightly flexed forward; "three-dimensional" correction is done in sequence: kyphotization (**a**), lateralization (**b**), and derotation (**c**). The first elastic band placed at the base of the ribs exerts a derotating force on the rib deformation typical of scoliotic condition.

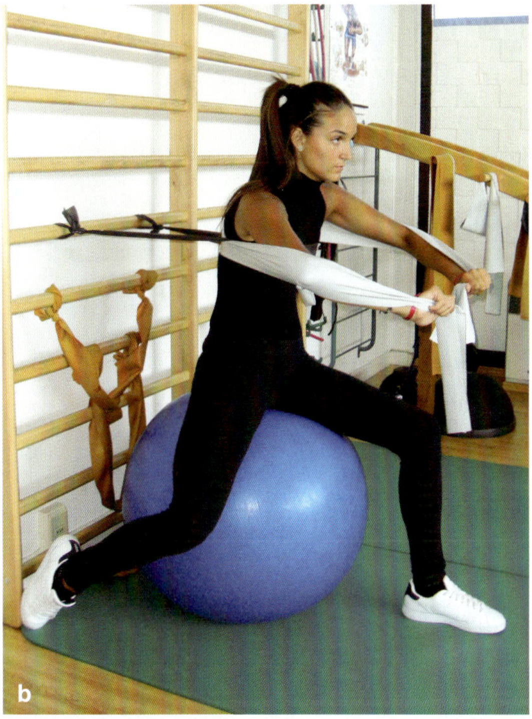

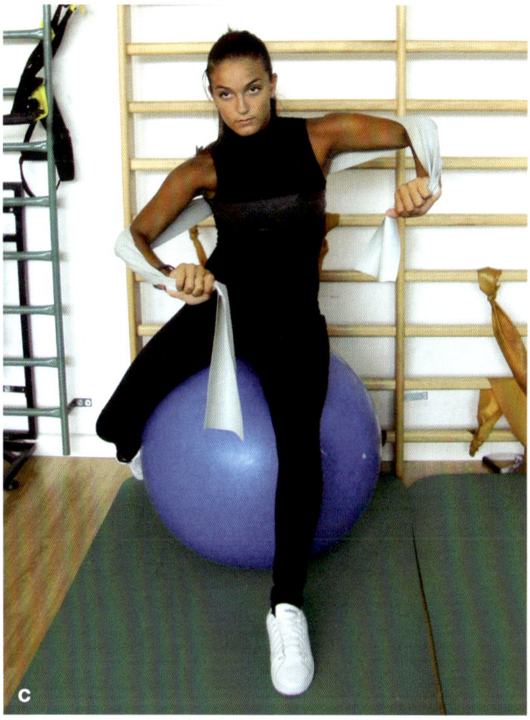

Group B

Group C

EXERCISE 5.44

Elastic Triad

The objective of this exercise is specific non-compensated three-dimensional dorsal correction.

Execution - The patient is in supine position in front of the wall bars. The cervical tract rests on an elastic band hooked around the fourth rung of the wall bars. The left arm grasps a second elastic band that wraps around the dorsal area of interest and generates traction and tension when brought away from the body, which reinforces the corrective movement. The legs, with a third band placed at the heels, compensate the lumbar counter-curve by rotating to the right. This exercise is prescribed only for experienced patients, due to its evident complexity and the simultaneous usage of several elastic bands.

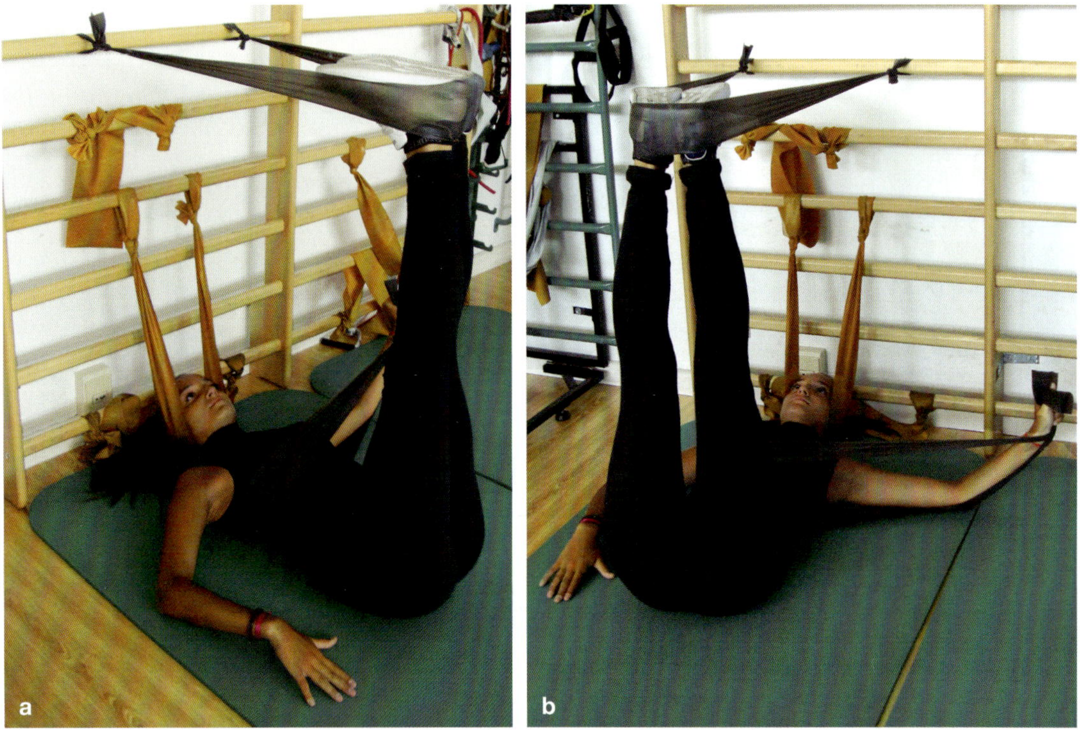

EXERCISE 5.45

Self-correction
This exercise is three-dimensional corrective, with particular attention paid to the containment of the lumbar curve.

Execution - An elastic band (black) is placed over the dorsal hump, and its two ends are gripped with the hands (the elbows remain wrapped within the band). A small weight is placed on the head to present a destabilizing load on the spinal column. A second elastic band (light gray) is placed to contain any left lumbar compensatory curve.

The knees are slightly flexed, then the trunk is flexed forward and three-dimensional correction is performed by pulling the elastic band with the left arm. It may be effective to squeeze a rhythmic gymnastics ball between the knees in order to favor greater lumbopelvic stabilization.

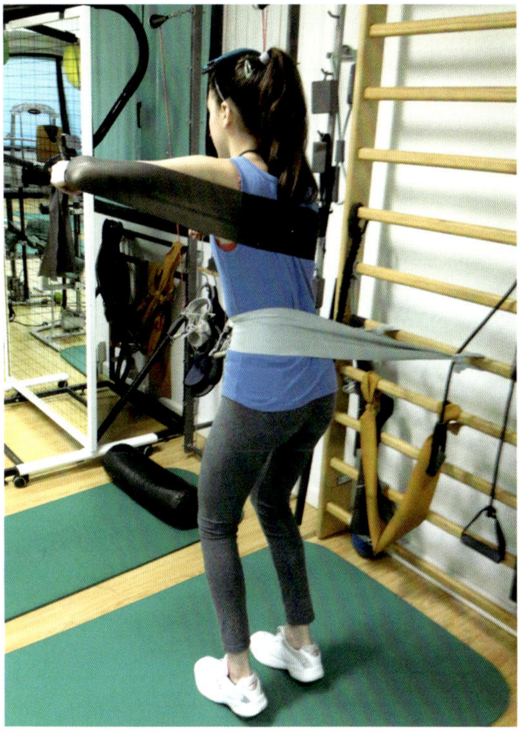

Group B

Group C

EXERCISE 5.46

Self-correction

This exercise is three-dimensional corrective, with particular attention paid to the containment of the lumbar curve.

Execution - The patient is positioned, as shown in the image, near the wall bars, with the right knee on the ground. An elastic band (black) is placed over the dorsal hump, and the two ends are grasped with the hands. Correction of the right dorsal hump is performed by providing a greater force with the left arm and seeking three-dimensional correction.

The gray elastic band, anchored to the wall bars at the level of the left dorsolumbar hump, contains any compensatory curve (left dorsolumbar).

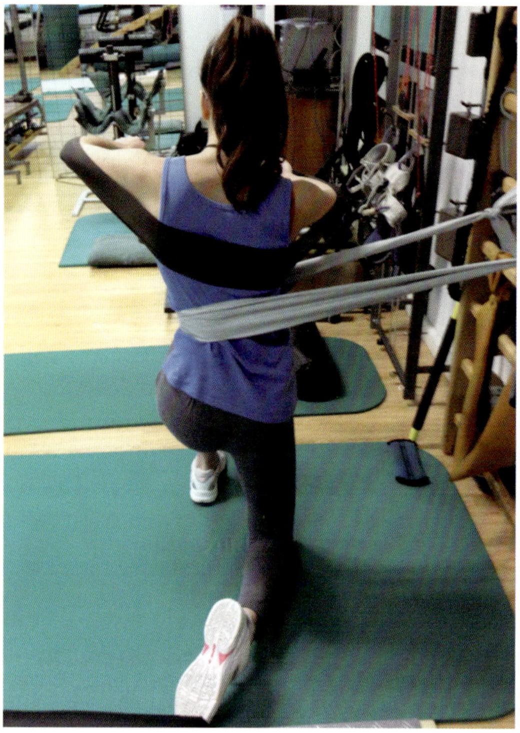

EXERCISE 5.47

Self-correction
This exercise is three-dimensional corrective, with particular attention paid to the containment of the lumbar curve.

Execution - Patient is in the prone position on the convex ladder. The gray elastic band is positioned over the right dorsal hump. Both ends of the elastic band are held with the left hand, which also grips a rung of the ladder. The left elbow must remain within the elastic band to act as a lever.
Both of the legs execute slight movement to the left in order to contain the left dorsolumbar compensatory curve. A rhythmic gymnastics ball placed between the knees facilitates greater lumbopelvic stabilization.
With the forehead resting on the ladder, the patient seeks kyphotization. Then, the right arm pushes on the gripped rung and the left arm pulls on it, favoring correction and progressively seeking lateralization and derotation.
Breathing, as always, happens in two stages: brief inhalation in preparation of the exercise; slow and prolonged exhalation maintained for the entire duration of the correction.

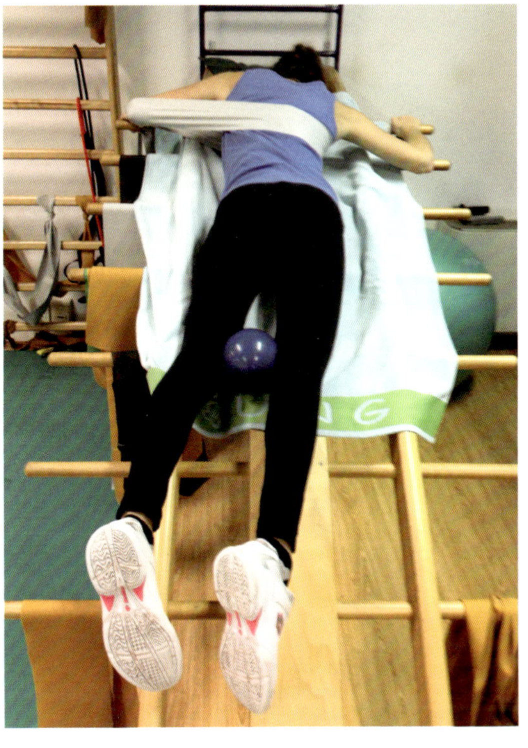

6

Dysmorphism at Full Skeletal Development

When working with patients who have dysmorphism at full skeletal development, the therapeutic indications and the approach begin with the sensitization of the patient to the possibility of improvement both aesthetically and with regards to pain. When approaching exercises, pain should always be avoided.

The exercises proposed involve:

- abdominal, paravertebral, and upper and lower limb strengthening and spinal stabilization exercises;
- stretching exercises for contracted muscles: psoas, ischiocrural, pectoral, and anti-gravitational muscles;
- respiratory exercises;
- development of coordinative abilities;
- exercises for the improvement of proprioceptive and exteroceptive perception (these have the function of providing stimuli that may improve the body scheme);
- exercises that reduce pain in general while improving the functionality of the areas of the body involved;
- core stability exercises.

On the other hand, it is prudent to avoid spinal mobilization exercises, because greater flexibility may, over time, promote worsening of the scoliotic curve. For avoiding pain, mobility is, however, useful for extraspinal joints that act as a release from endogenous and exogenous stress placed on the vertebral column.

Core stability (stabilization of the nucleus) exercises play a very important role in the prevention and treatment of vertebral pathologies, above all with adult scoliosis. Core stability concerns the ability to enact and maintain good motor control, particularly in the lumbopelvic area, so as to create a solid structural basis. The muscles activated during core stability are, particularly, the straight, transverse, external and internal oblique abdominal muscles, the quadratus lumborum, and the dorsal muscles. The deep muscles, namely the transverse, multifidus, internal oblique, paraspinal muscles, and the muscles of the pelvic floor, are the key to active support of the lumbar column and thus to stabilization of the area itself.

EXERCISE 6.1

Corrective

Three-dimensional dorsal correction and containment of the lumbar curve.

Execution - With the patient seated on a Swiss ball, with the ends of the elastic band anchored to the left of the body, the patient pulls with the left arm higher than the right arm so as to favor three-dimensional correction. The legs are positioned so as to contain any lumbar counter-curve. This exercise is also indicated for painful adult scoliosis.

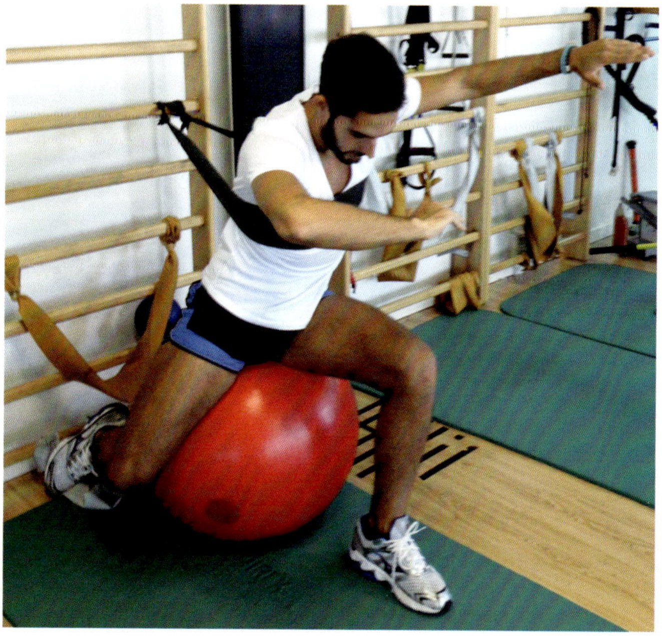

EXERCISE 6.2

Stretching of the Psoas

The objective of this exercise is to progressively stretch the iliopsoas muscle by distancing the origin of the muscle (T12-L5) from its insertion on the lesser trochanter, thus creating sarcomeres in series (if the psoas muscle is found to be shortened in the evaluation test, this exercise may be very useful).

Execution - Two bands are placed respectively on the suprapatellar region and on the dorsum of the foot; the leg remains slightly lifted off the floor. It is important that the angle between the thigh and the trunk remains open by keeping of the trunk extended with the aid of some device (for example, two batons).

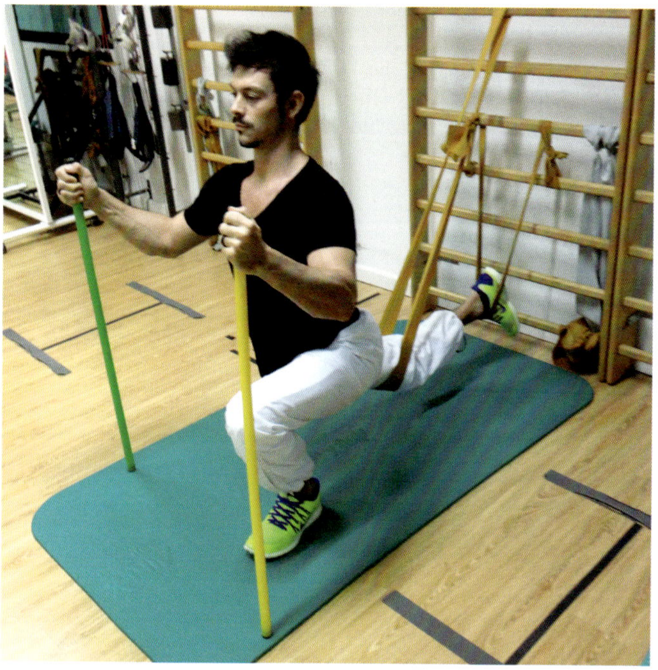

EXERCISE 6.3

Decontracting

This exercise, performed with the Rovatti Balance, is highly decontracting for the cervicodorsal tract.

Execution - The head rests in a neutral position on the elastic band so as to maintain a situation of maximum relaxation of the cervical tract (the head should remain about 5-20 mm from the floor). The legs rest on a Swiss ball in order to obtain total relaxation.

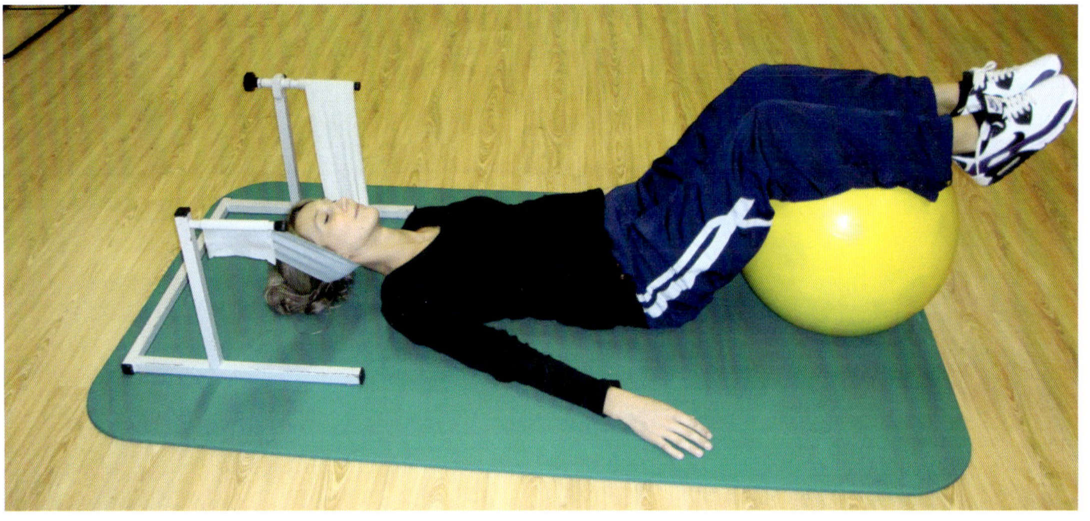

Rovatti Balance: This device is a structure on which an elastic band is laid and kept stable with the desired tension (adjustable). It is used to fully decontract the cervical and dorsal tracts (a trademark of the Rovatti Plan®).

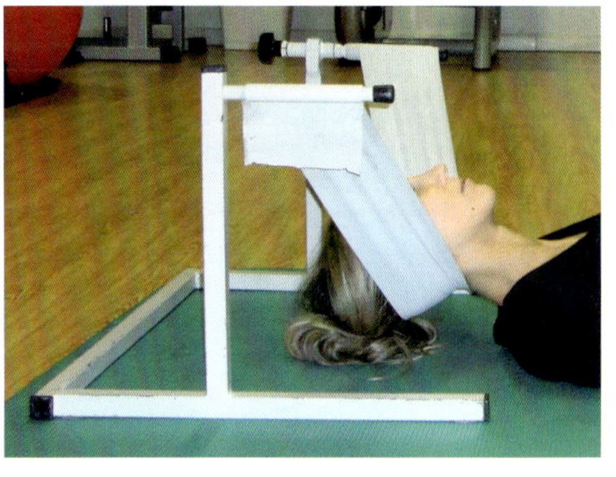

Group D

EXERCISE 6.4

Lumbosacral Unloading in Flexion

Execution - Using two elastic bands of maximum strength (maximum density and resistance) hooked onto a high rung of the wall bars, a Swiss ball is placed under the gluteus. The pelvis is slid backwards in order to obtain tension relief and unloading of the dorsal-lumbar-sacral components.

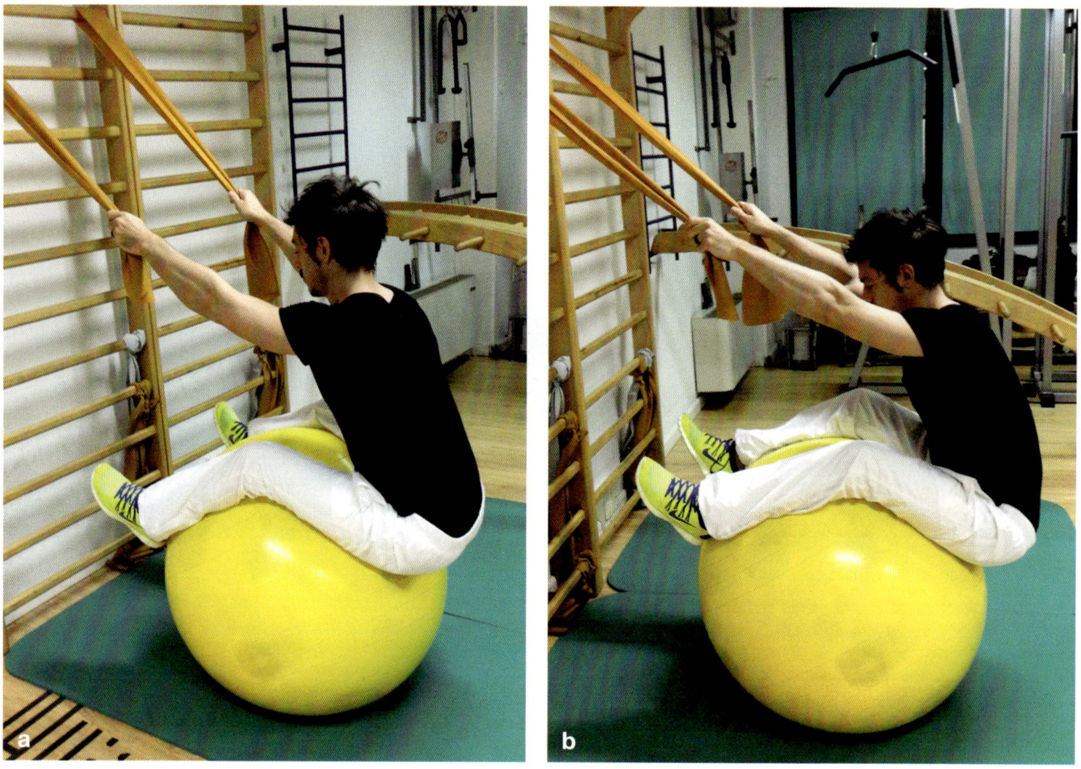

EXERCISE 6.5

Lumbar Unloading in Extension

This exercise is indicated for dorsolumbar kyphosis and radiculopathies in the lower limbs.

Execution - The patient keeps the ends of two elastic bands hooked onto a high rung of the wall bars. The patient stretches out on two Swiss balls: one of greater diameter positioned at the dorsal area, and one of smaller diameter at the posterior area of the legs. The patient slowly lowers the pelvis toward the floor in order to obtain decontraction of the extended lumbar region maintaining the physiological curves.

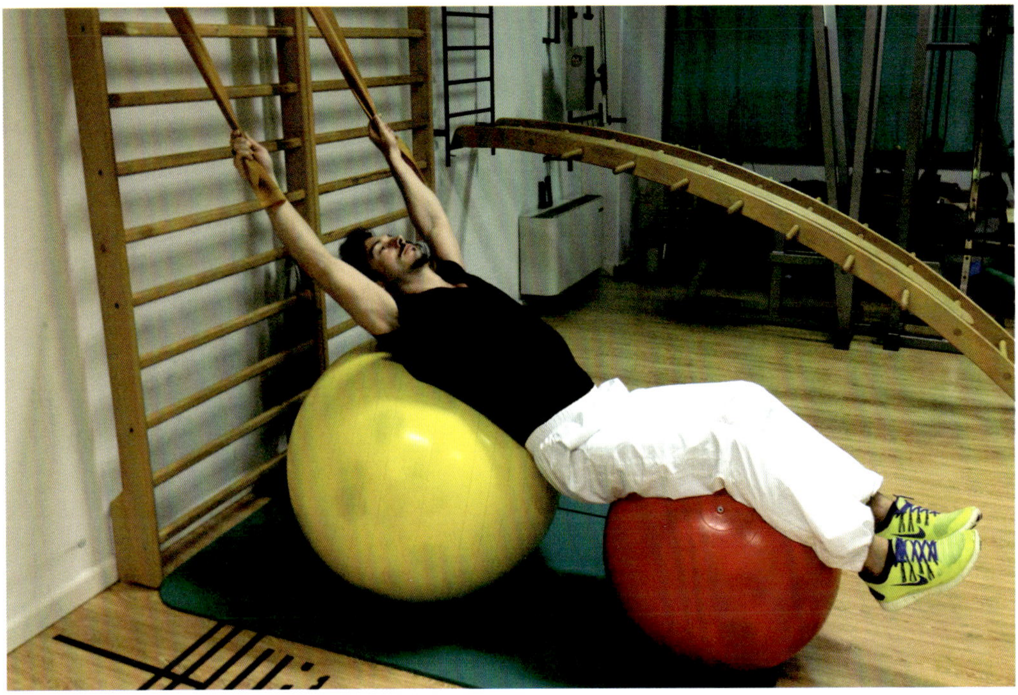

Group D

EXERCISE 6.6

Abdominal Strengthening and Stabilization of the Spine

Execution - The patient is in the supine position with the legs lifted off the ground and at right angles: a medicine ball is held between the knees and the head is slightly lifted. The elastic band, held with the hands and fixed to the wall bars, is pulled (**a**); at the same time, pivoting on the fixed point of the hands, slight correction (**b**) is performed on the three spatial planes (kyphotization, lateralization, and derotation).

a, The male subject uses an elastic band of greater resistance;
b, the female subject uses an elastic band of lesser resistance.

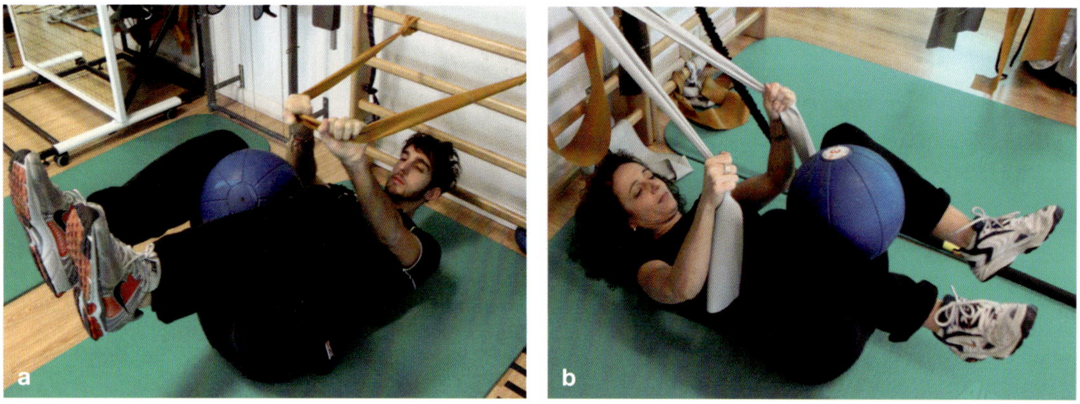

EXERCISE 6.7

Core Stability

This exercise is for abdominal reinforcement of the lower limbs and the gluteus muscles, maintaining lumbopelvic stability.

Execution - The elastic band is placed at the abdominopelvic region with the legs resting on a Swiss ball; the pelvis is lifted against resistance.

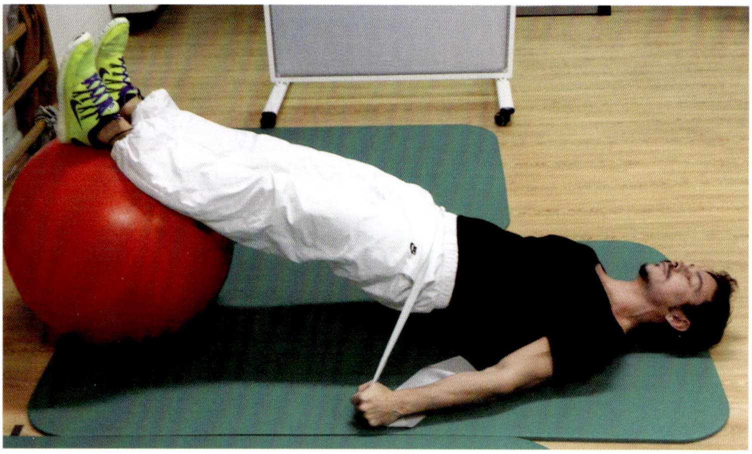

EXERCISE 6.8

Passive Antalgic Stretching

This exercise is performed with the *Ro-Plan Fly*, a piece of equipment conceived and patented by the Rovatti Plan®.

Execution - A girth is positioned at the pelvic region, held by several elastic bands of maximum resistance (these must be calibrated according to the person's weight). The feet are set in starting block-like position on a graduated bar, and the entire body is lowered forward in a natural manner (**a**). With the knees semi-flexed, the body is balanced in order to obtain strongly antalgic passive stretching (**b**). Once in a position of total vertebral unloading and tension relief of the paravertebral muscles, the patient enacts correction on the three spatial planes, favoring lateralization and derotation with the left arm extended to the left (**c**, **d**).

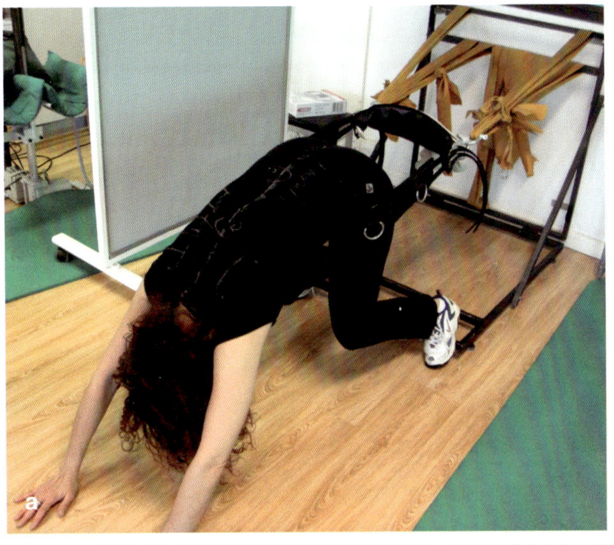
a

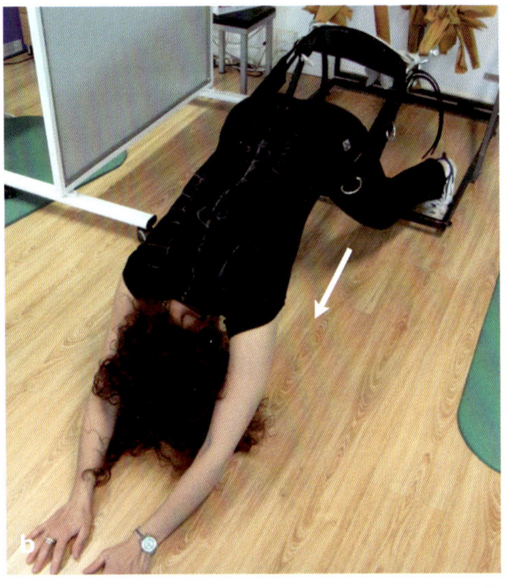
b

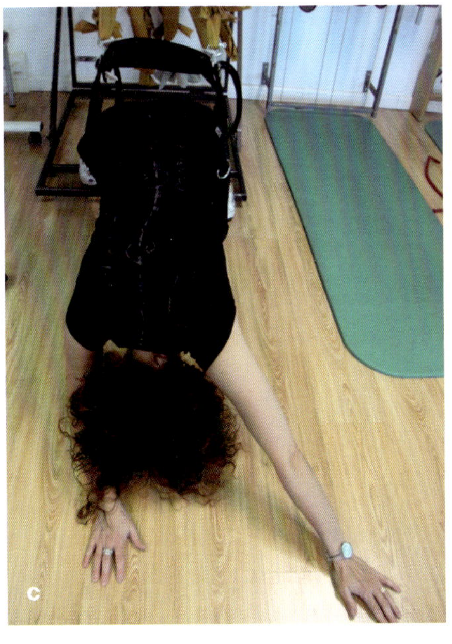
c

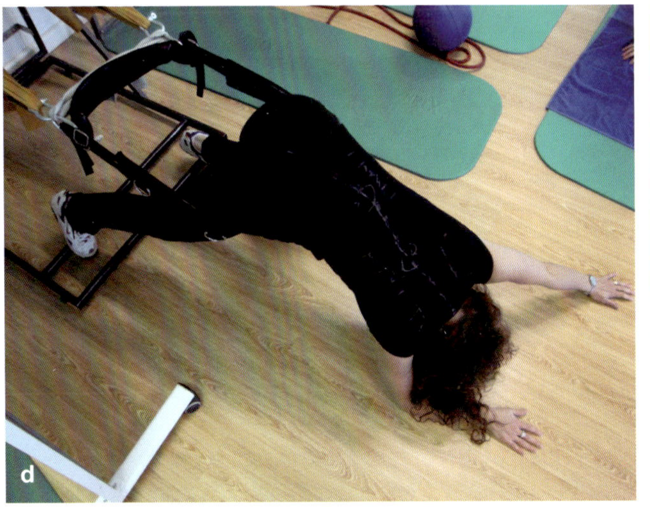
d

Group D

EXERCISE 6.9

Core Stability

Supine-position lifting of the gluteus muscles to intensify lumbopelvic stabilization.

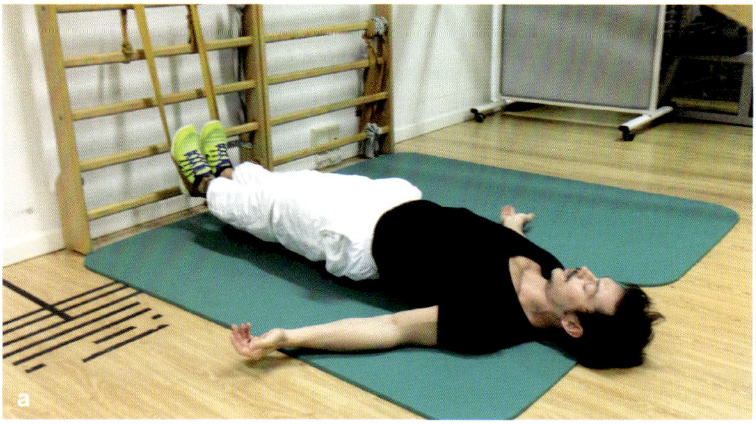

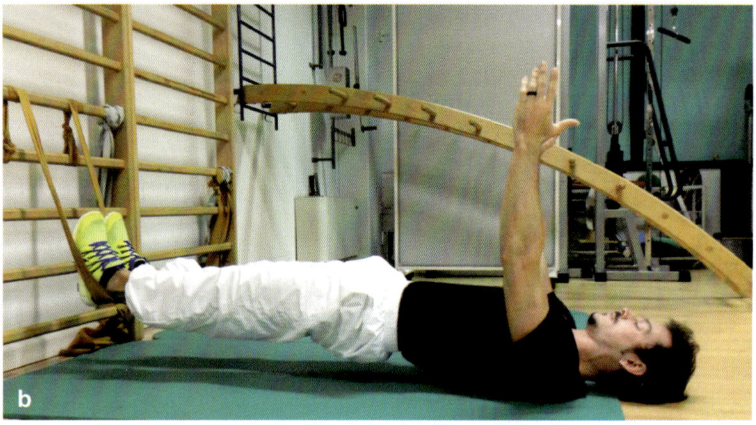

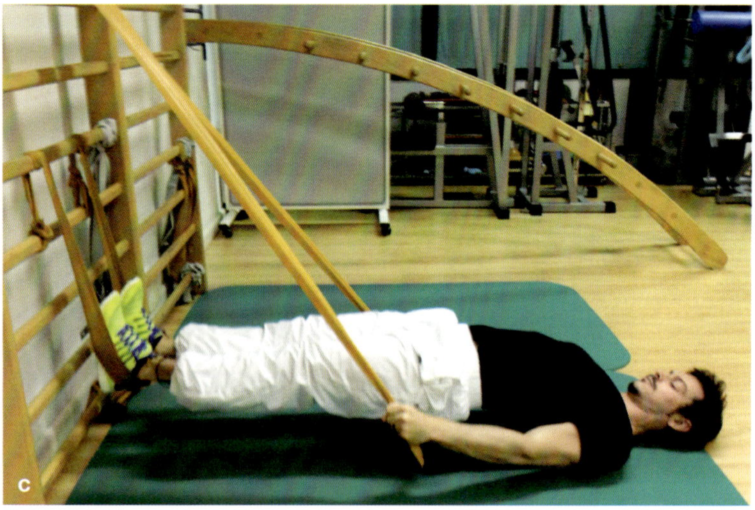

Execution - With the patient in the supine position (**a**), the heels, which are lifted, are positioned on the elastic band; the gluteus muscles are lifted, maintaining lumbopelvic control (retroversion of the pelvis; lumbopelvic stabilization; **b**).

Variant - In order to increase the degree of lumbopelvic stabilization, two elastic bands, attached to a high rung of the wall bars, are gripped (**c**).

EXERCISE 6.10

Core Stability

Activation of the core with the legs lifted in the supine position. Objective: improve control and performance of the abdominal muscles by maintaining the neutral position of the spine.

Execution - The subject is in the supine position, with a baton or a pen placed behind the lumbar region (**a**) to aid in the maintenance of the neutral position of the lumbar tract (there should be neither too much pressure nor too much separation). The core (nucleus) is activated by simultaneously pulling the elastic band (**b**); next, the lower limbs, flexed at 90 degrees, are lifted, and their distance from the body is adjusted based on contact with or separation from the baton under the lumbar region (**c**).

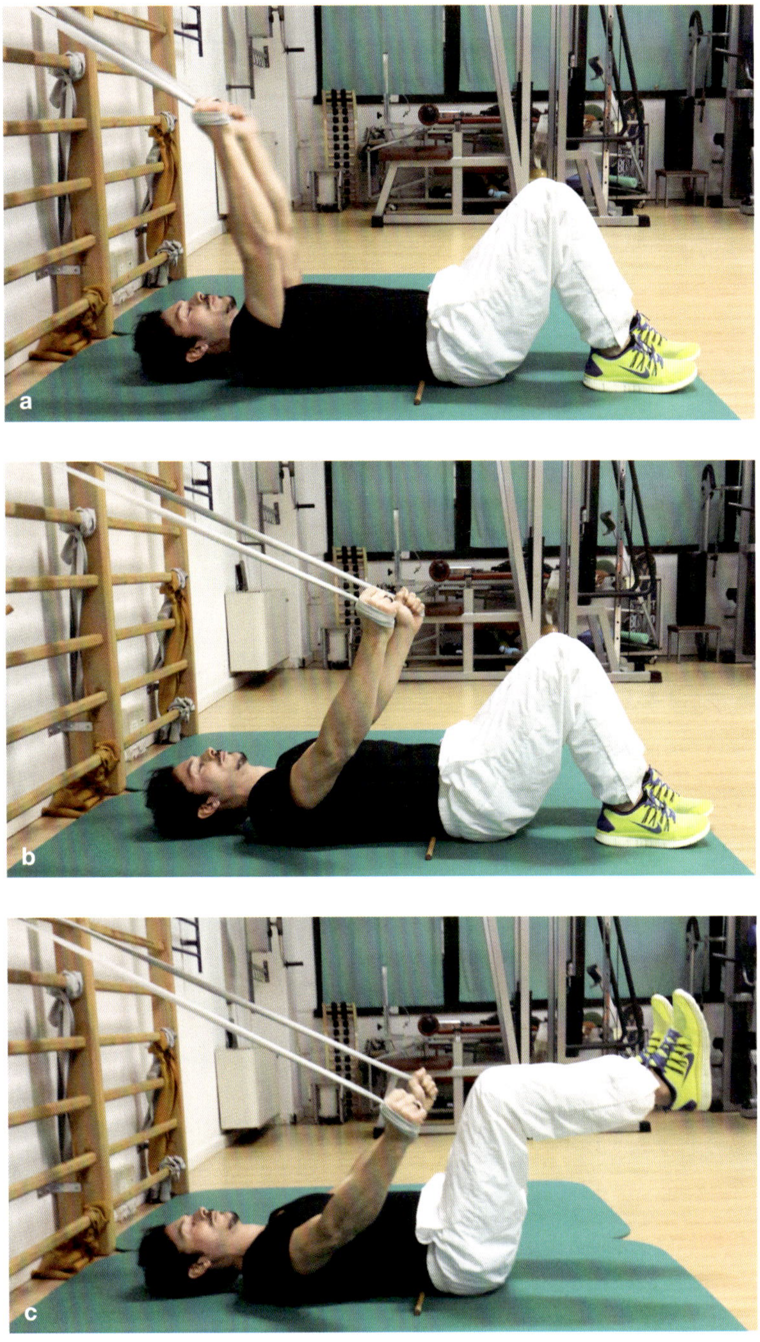

Group D

EXERCISE 6.11

Core Stability

Stabilization of the core from the quadruped position. This exercise has the aim of maintaining an optimal activation of the core by paying particular attention to the oblique abdominal muscles (which have the role of preventing rotation of the pelvis) in the presence of a destabilizing element (elastic band). It thus improves the performance of the abdominal muscles, control of the spine, balance, and control of the pelvis in preventing rotation.

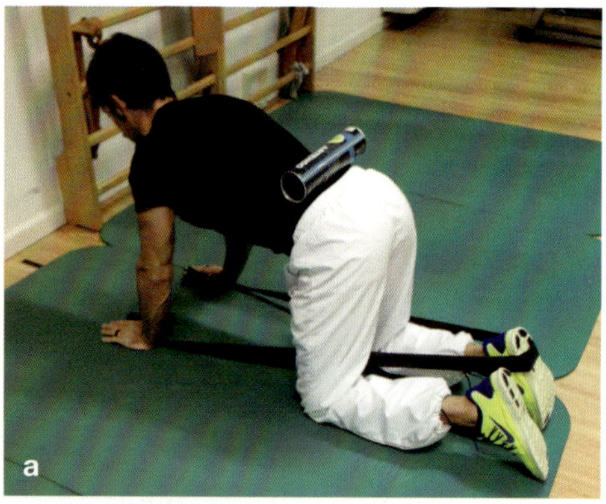
a

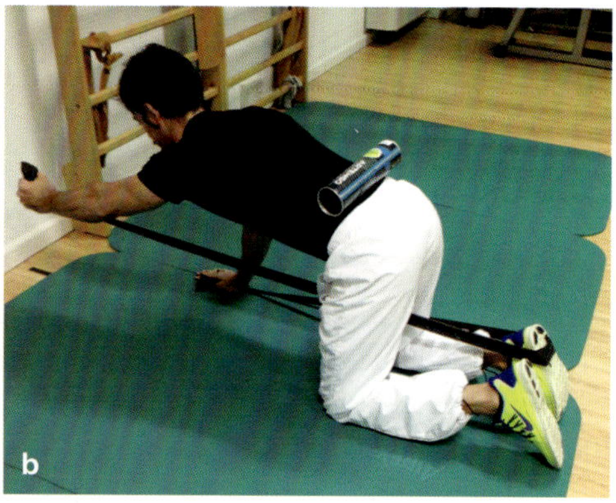
b

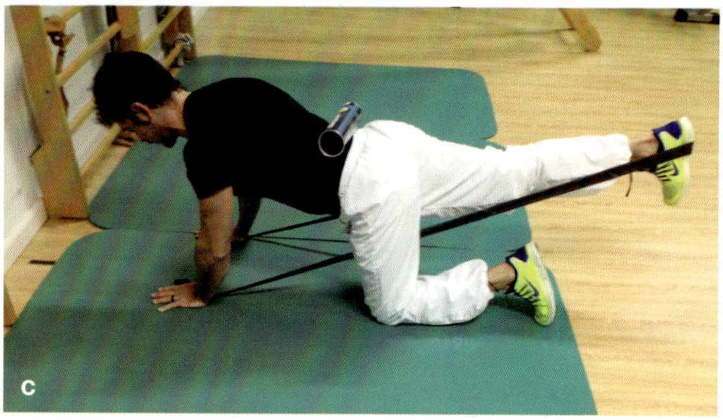
c

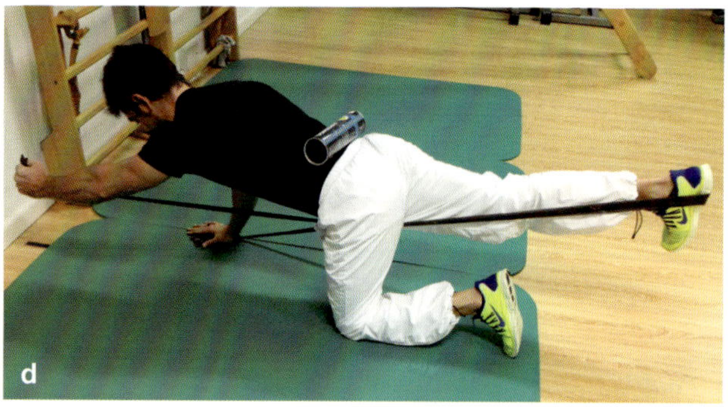
d

Execution - The patient gets into a quadruped position, aligning body segments (knees in line with femurs and hands in line with shoulders) and distributing the weight over the four points of support (**a**). An elastic band is fixed behind one foot and its ends are gripped with the hands; the back is kept in a neutral position and the core (nucleus) is activated, particularly the oblique muscles, in order to avoid rotation of the pelvis during execution. The exercise is initiated by flexing the upper limb holding the elastic (**b**). If the exercise is properly performed, it proceeds to the second phase, with the lower limb being extended against the elastic's resistance and the position being held (**c**). Only when the patient is able to maintain the position without compensations or rotations should they move on to the third phase (**d**). Each of the positions is held for at least 10 seconds.

In order to avoid breakdowns in posture during the execution of this exercise, it is useful to place a cylindrical support at the lumbar region (a plastic bottle may also be used) that will not fall if the proper position (neutral position) is maintained.

EXERCISE 6.12

Core Stability

Activation of the core in quadruped position with a Swiss ball. Objective: keep the body stable using the core with an activation element (Swiss ball).

Execution - A Swiss ball rests against a wall or wall bars; an elastic band is wrapped around the gluteus muscles. The patient gets into the quadruped position with the gluteus muscles in contact with the ball; the hands (gripping the ends of the elastic) are on the floor (**a**). The neutral position of the spine is held, and the ball is compressed with the gluteus muscles (**b**) in order to achieve strong activation of the abdominal muscles by counterforce. Finally, the upper limb (with the elastic in the hand) is flexed (**c**) and held in an unchanged position for 10 seconds, avoiding rotation.

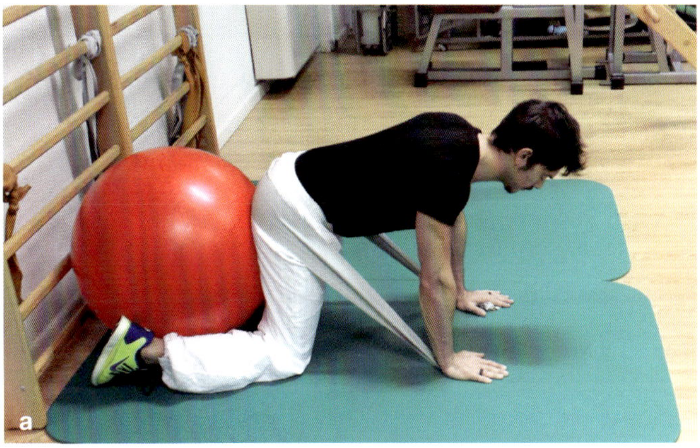

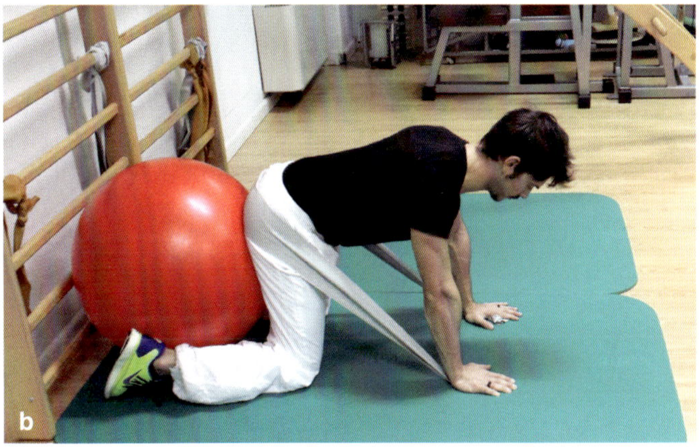

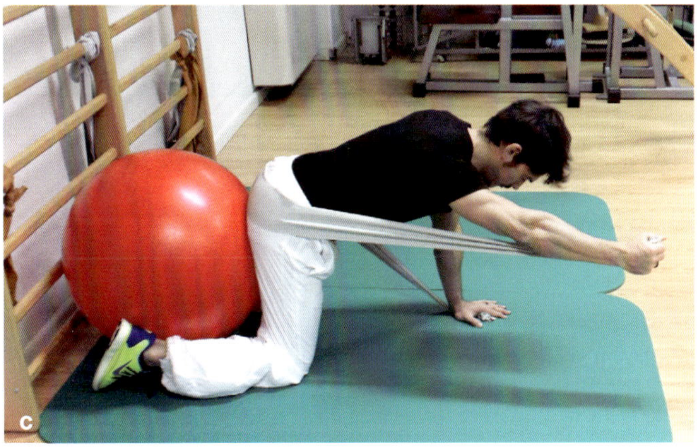

Group D

EXERCISE 6.13

Core Stability

Lumbopelvic stabilization, from the supine position, on a cylinder.

Execution - In the supine position on a rubber cylinder, with an elastic band wrapped around the wall bars (**a**), the elastic band held by the arms is pulled (**b**); the patient avoids losing spinal contact with the cylinder. The patient maintains balance and reinforces lumbopelvic stabilization by lifting first one leg (**c**) and then the other (**d**).

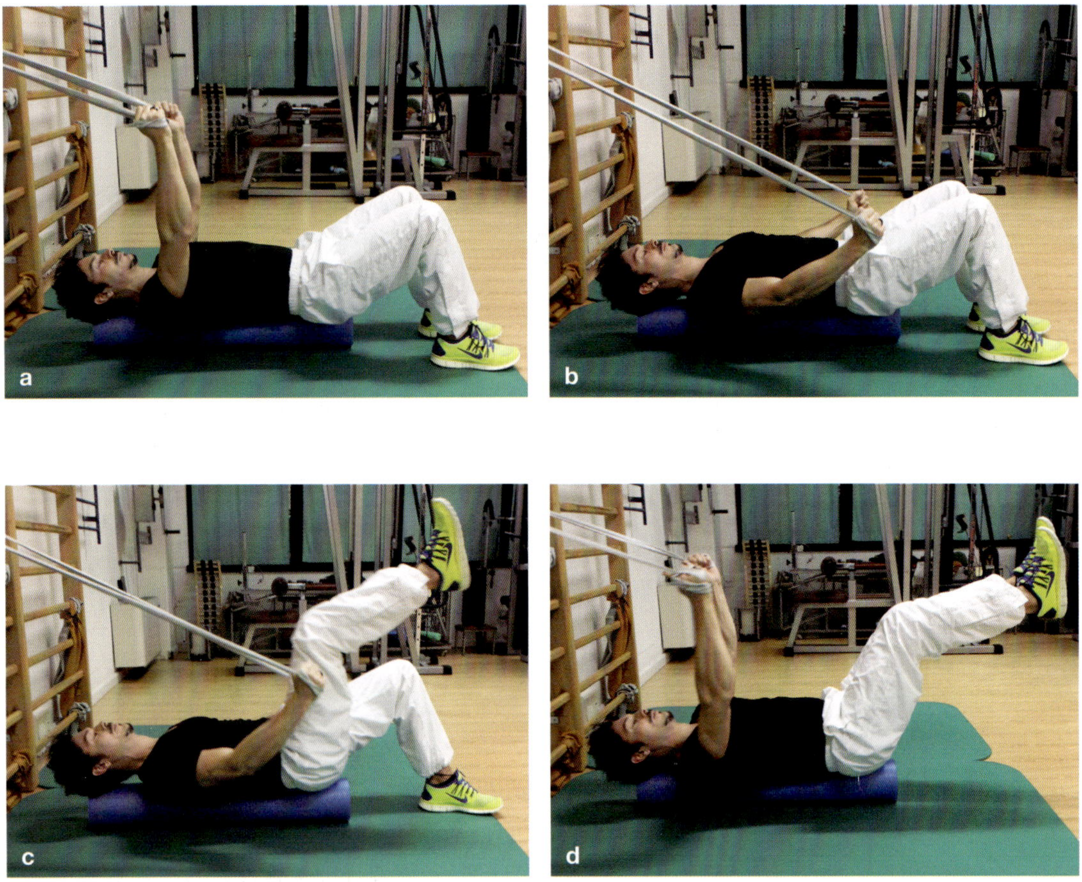

EXERCISE 6.14

Core Stability

Stabilization while standing upright with a baton used as a rotating destabilization element. Objective: reduce rotation acting upon spinal column, maintaining the body stable.

Execution - An elastic band is anchored to the end of a baton and to a wall bar (asymmetrical destabilizing action). With the patient standing upright, the body is held in line and the arms are brought forward, keeping them tensed and gripping the baton. Next, the leg opposite the fulcrum of the elastic band is lifted to 90 degrees (**a**) while keeping the abdominal muscles active and avoiding rotation. After this first level of the exercise is achieved, the patient moves onto the next level (**b**) by flexing the lower limb homolateral to the fulcrum of the elastic. At the end, the fulcrum is moved to the opposite side and the exercise is repeated.

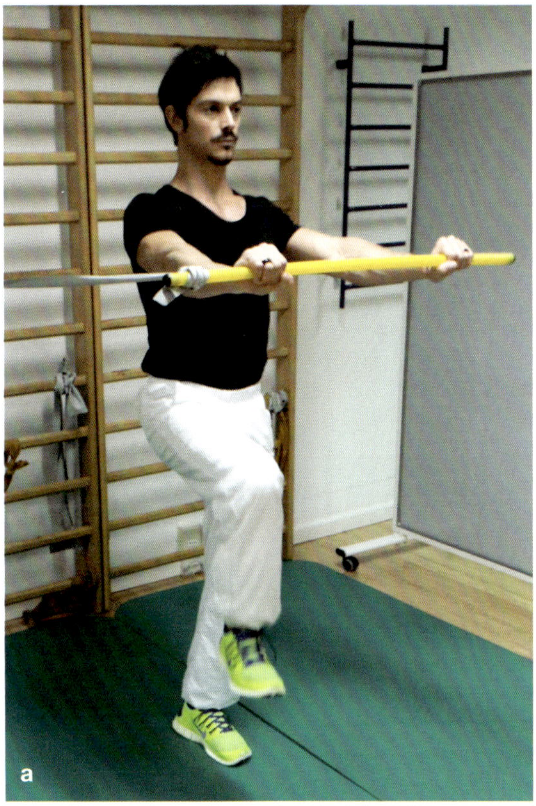
a

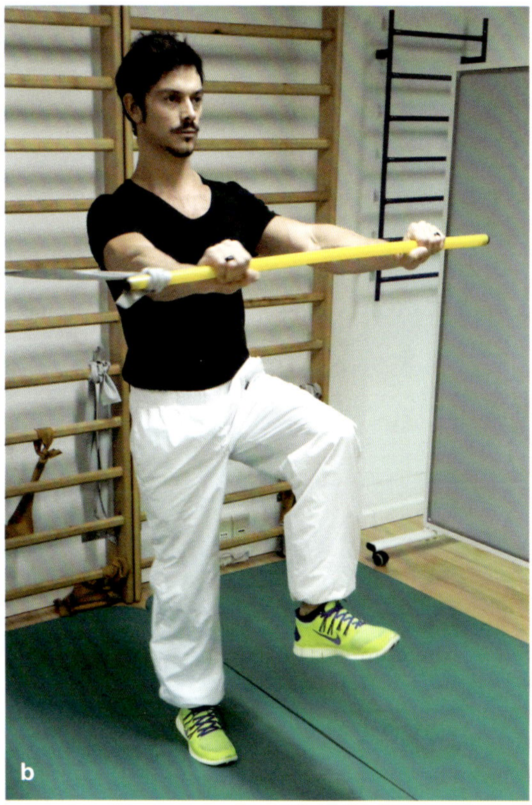
b

Group D

EXERCISE 6.15

Core stability

Activation of the core with active straight leg raise (ASLRs). The objective of the exercise is to recreate the proper core activation sequence via pre-activation provided by the extension of the upper limbs. It also develops skill in separating the lower extremities via the flexion of a limb and stabilization on the ground (extension of the opposite limb with activation of the gluteus muscles).

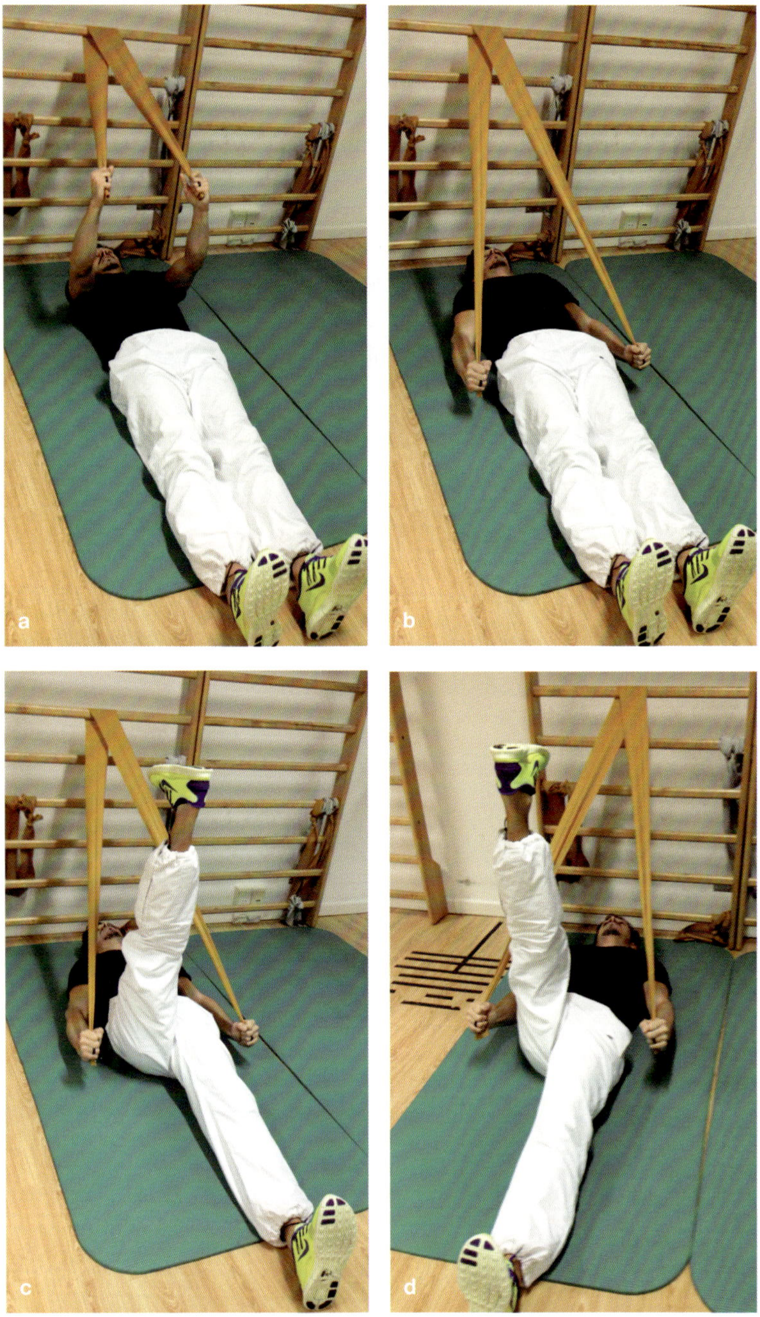

Execution - From the supine starting position (**a**), the patient executes an activation sequence structured as follows: extend the upper limbs and pull the elastic band (**b**); lift the stretched lower limb without breaking composure and maintaining the alignment of the lower limbs and the feet, sustaining tension for 2-3 seconds with the feet raised (**c**); lower the leg (**d**) and repeat 6-8 times before changing the limb. After having lowered the lower limb, it is imperative that the elastic tension be released and reactivated for each repetition.

EXERCISE 6.16

Core Stability

Activation of the core with the patient standing upright. The objective of the exercise is to recreate the proper core activation sequence via pre-activation provided by the extension of the upper limbs.

Execution - With the patient standing upright and bringing the posture as close as possible to the physiological state of spinal curvature, the patient extends the upper limbs against the resistance of the elastic (**a**) and performs 90-degree flexion of the hip with the knee bent and with the lower supporting limb kept extended due to the activation of the gluteus muscles (**b**).

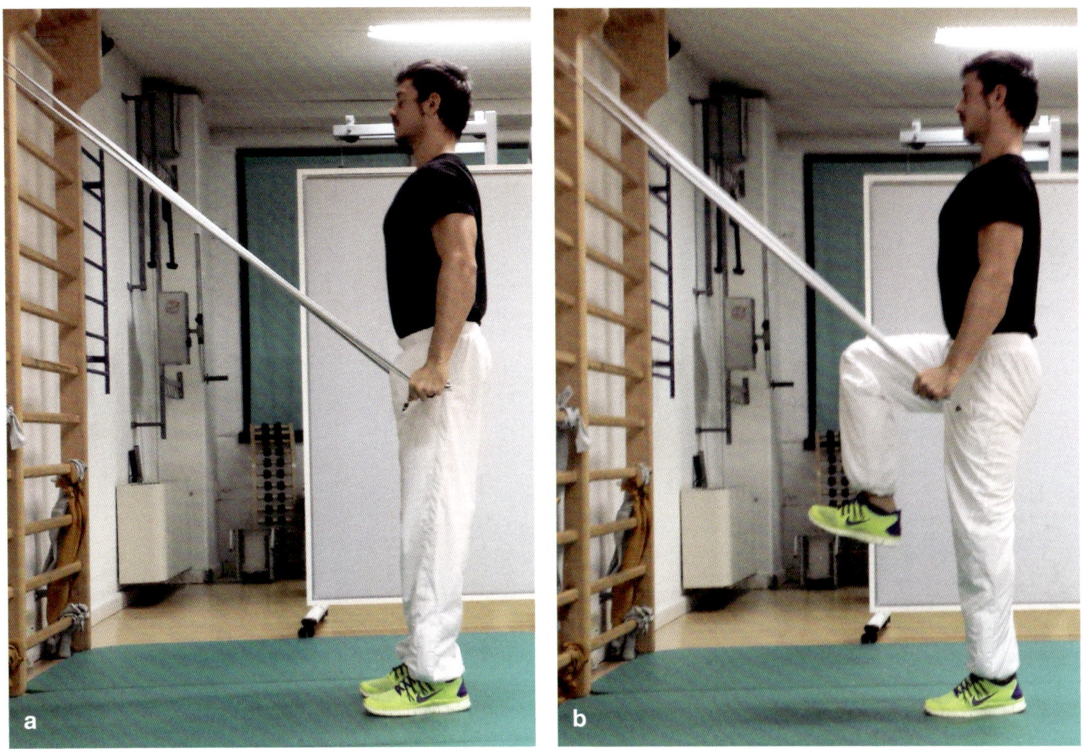

Group D

EXERCISE 6.17

Core Stability

Plank with elastic in the hands, in order to increase the holding ability of the lumbopelvic stabilizing muscles.

Execution - From the quadruped position, the patient grips the two ends of one or two elastic bands anchored to wall bars (moderate tension is needed in order to sustain the weight of the body). The patient brings the body gradually into tension by stabilizing the trunk to the point at which the patient succeeds in maintaining core activation without causing negative tensions (interrupting the lines of the body) at the lumbar area or the back.

This exercise may be performed both with the wall bars behind the shoulders (**a**, **b**) or facing the wall bars (**c**, **d**, **e**).

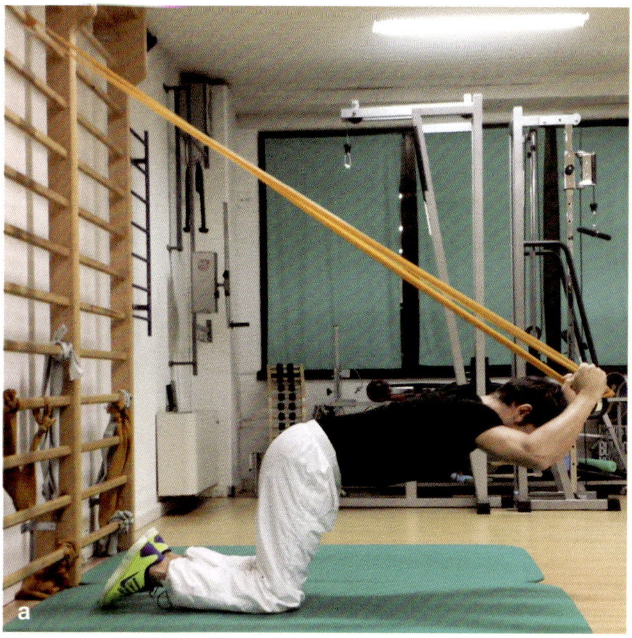
a

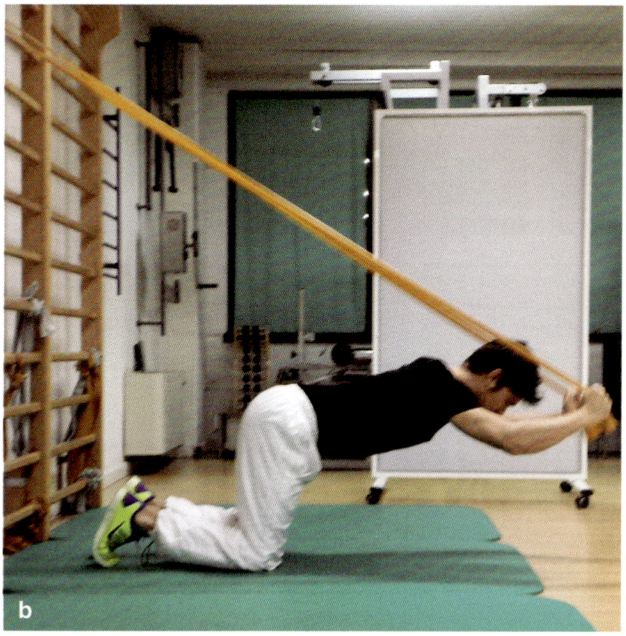
b

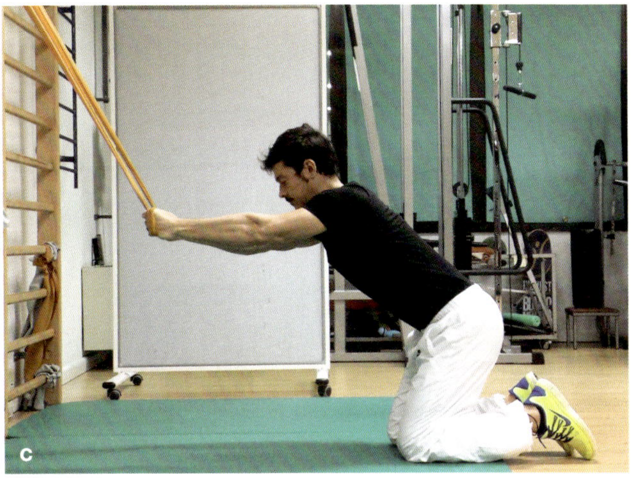

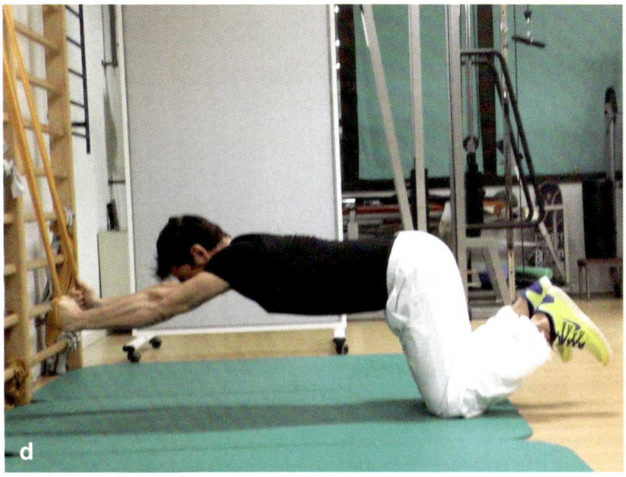

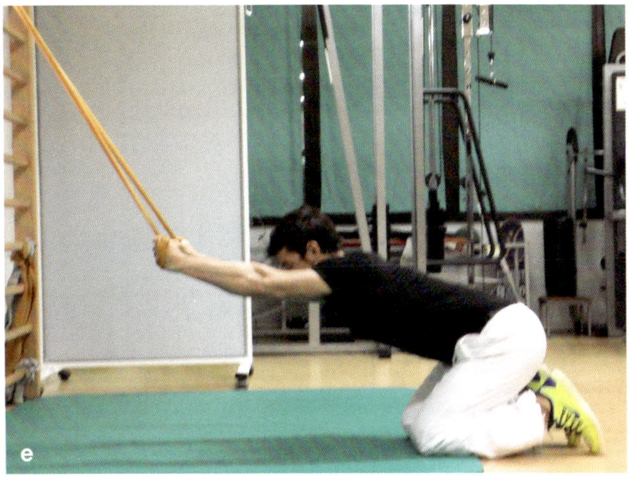

Group D

EXERCISE 6.18

Core Stability

Plank with destabilization of the dorsum of the feet, in order to increase the holding ability of the lumbopelvic stabilizing muscles with a destabilizing element.

Execution - The subject rests the elbows on the ground in a holding position and sets the dorsum of both feet on a high-tension elastic band. The patient brings the spinal curve into physiological state and holds this position for at least 10-20 seconds, activating the core (**a**, **b**).

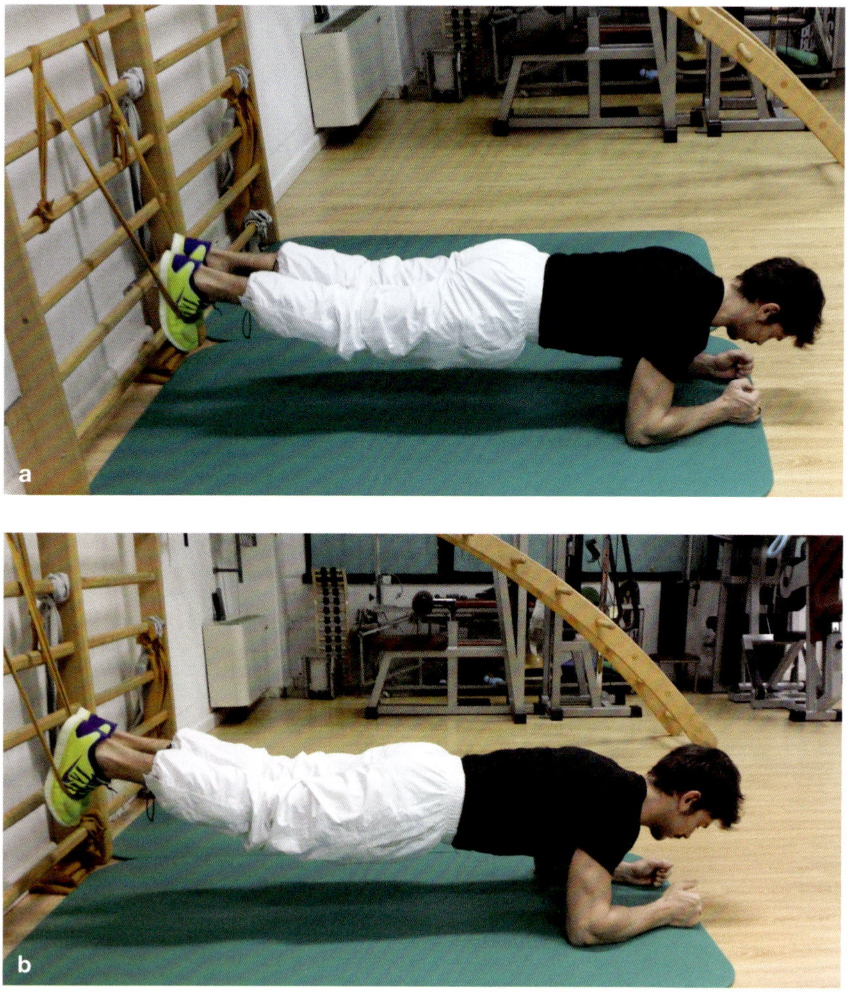

EXERCISE 6.19

Core Stability

Side bridge with elastic counter-force. Objective: maintain the linearity of body segments in the side bridge position with the action of external destabilizing forces, thus increasing the performance of the lateral fasciae of the core (nucleus).

Execution - The subject is positioned on the side; an elastic band is wrapped around the back, positioned under the forearm and held with the hands. The body is lifted with the feet together and the forearm on the ground, keeping body segments aligned. In the first phase (**a**), the upper limb is stretched upward for at least 10 seconds. Then, the arm is brought frontally (**b**) so as to obtain an anterior-posterior counter-force. Once a proper quality of execution of the exercise is achieved, a soft elastic band is added between the two feet and the abduction of the lower limbs is incorporated into both phases. This position is held for 10 seconds (**c**, **d**).

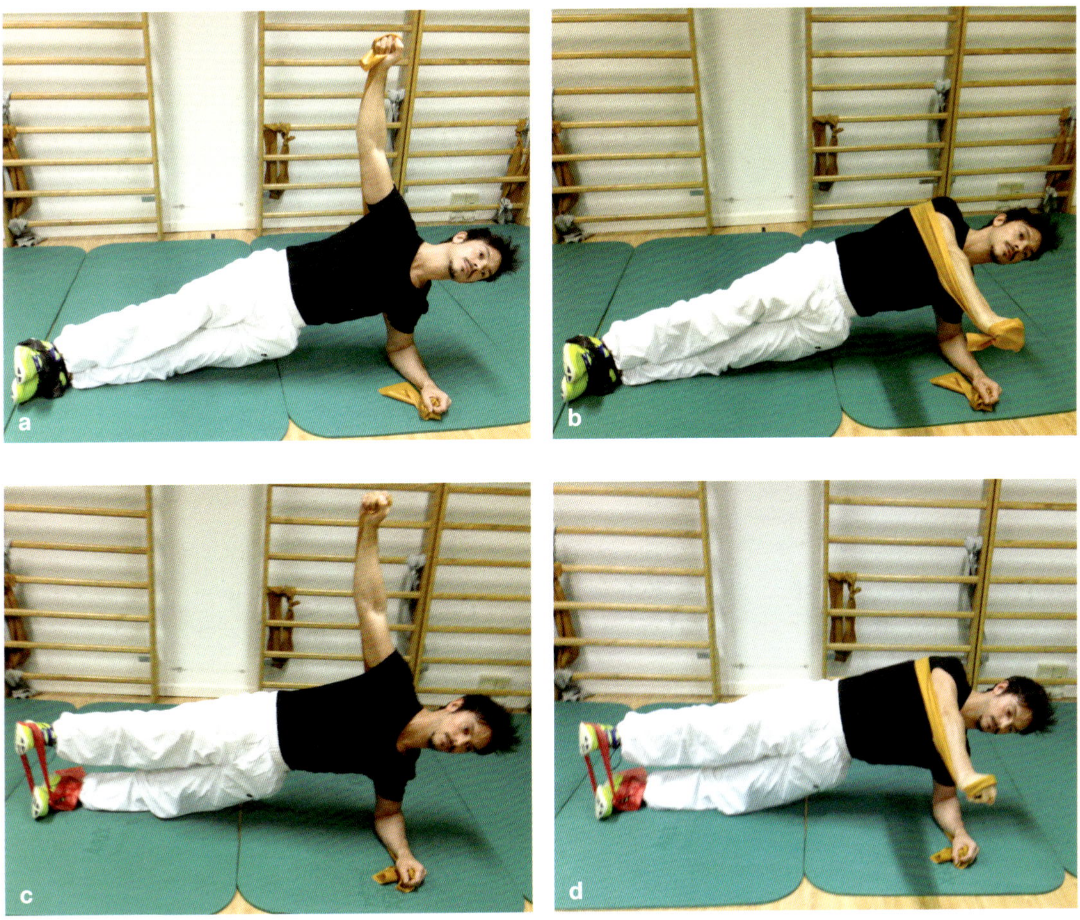

Bibliography

Antonini G, Negrini S, Cararziona R, Marinoni E. Evolutività della scoliosi. In: Monografie Gruppo di Studio della Scoliosi. Vigevano: GSS, 2000.

Badelon B, Boitier C. Les tractions vertébrales. (33° Numéro specialisè). In: Encyclopedie médico-chirurgicale Kinésitherapie Rééducation fonctionnelle. Paris: Edition Technicques, 1985.

Becchetti S. Diagnosi e prognosi della scoliosi: ultime acquisizioni. Le Scienze Motorie 1993; 2: 11-9.

Biot B, Mollon G, Ollier M, Stortz M. Attitudes scoliotiques. (48° Numéro specialisè). In: Encyclopedie médico-chirurgicale, Kinésitherapie Rééducation fonctionnelle. Paris: Edition Technicques, 1992.

Capurso U, Marini I, Alessandri Bonetti G. I disordini cranio-mandibolari: fisioterapia speciale stomatognatica. Bologna: Edizioni Martina, 1996.

Chahuneau J. Techniques de rèèducation respiratoire. (31° Numéro specialisè). In: Encyclopedie médico-chirurgicale Kinésitherapie Rééducation fonctionnelle. Paris: Edition Technicques, 1984.

Charrière L, Roy J. Kinésithérapie des déviations latérales du rachis. II edition. Paris: Masson, 1973.

Charrière L, Roy J. Les déviations antéro-postérieures du rachis. (12° Numéro specialisè). In: Encyclopedie médico-chirurgicale Kinésitherapie Rééducation fonctionnelle. Paris: Edition Technicques, 1978.

Clarkson HM. Valutazione cinesiologica. Milano: Edi.Ermes, 1991.

Corigliano A, Ceppatelli S, Dafra C, Mencarelli M. Il dolore nella grave scoliosi dell'adulto. In: P. Sibilla, S. Negrini (eds). Il trattamento della lombalgia. Milano: Edi.Ermes, 1996; pagg. 35-9.

Costanzo G, Cellocco P, Ranieri A. Corsetti per scoliosi secondo le diverse scuole terapeutiche: prescrizione, costruzione, collaudo ed esercizi specifici. Stato dell'arte nel trattamento conservativo delle scoliosi. In: Rachide e riabilitazione multidisciplinare. Terzo Evidence-Based Meeting, Vigevano: GSS, 2007.

Cristofanilli M. Nuove metodiche chinesiterapiche nella rieducazione delle scoliosi con tecniche basate sugli equilibri. Le Scienze Motorie 1990; 3: 32-8.

Cristofanilli MA. 1° Congresso società spagnola di fisioterapia. Barcellona, 1994.

Cunha HM, Cesarani A, Ciancaglini R, et al. Postura, occlusione, rachide: problematiche interdisciplinari. Bassano del Grappa: Edizioni C.P.A., 1992.

Daniels L, Worthingham C. Esercizi terapeutici, Roma: Verduci Editore, 1980.

Ducongè P. La scoliosi in età evolutiva. In: Atti del XIX Congresso GEKTS, Modena, 1991.

Ducongè P, Guilloux R. La scoliose aujourd'hui, la scoliose demain. Lyon: Groupe Europeen kinesitherapique travail scoliose (GEKTS),1992.

Efther G, Prau JP. Méthodes gymniques de rèeducation vertébrale. (45° Numéro specialisè). In: Encyclopedie médico-chirurgicale, Kinésitherapie Rééducation fonctionnelle. Paris: Edition Technicques, 1991.

Fusco MA. Trattato di Posturologia. Vol. 1° Introduzione alla posturologia. Avellino: VIP Servizi Edizioni, 2004.

Gans M. Méthodes gymniques de rèèducation vertebrale. (25° Numéro specialisè). In: Encyclopedie médico-chirurgicale, Kinésitherapie Rééducation fonctionnelle. Paris: Edition Technicques, 1981.

Greissing H, Zillo A. Zilgrei: come eliminare da soli il mal di schiena e i dolori da artrosi lombare. Milano: Mondadori, 1998.

Kapandji IA. Fisiologia articolare. Roma: Marrapese Editore, 1983.

Kos B. 1200 esercizi di ginnastica. Roma: Società Stampa Sportiva, 1973.

Mariotto F. Rieducazione psico-motoria e ginnastica ortopedica nelle alterazioni morfolofiche funzionali e strutturali. 2° edizione. Milano: Sperling&Kupfer,1974.
Massara G. Attualità in chinesiterapia. Roma: Edizioni Marrapese, 1991.
Mazzocco G. Chinesiologia itinerante. In: Atti del Convegno Nazionale UNC, Venezia 1985.
Negrini S, Sibilla P. Il peso degli zainetti scolastici. Un problema di salute pubblica? Milano: Fondazione Don Carlo Gnocchi, 2000.
Negrini S, Sibilla P. Le deformità vertebrali: stato dell'arte. Volume 1°, Vigevano: GSS, 2000.
Negrini S, Sibilla P. Le deformità vertebrali: stato dell'arte. Volume 2°, Vigevano: GSS, 2001.
Niquet G, Bierry L, Bierry M. Controindicazioni alla pratica sportiva. Roma: Marrapese Editore, 1982.
Perdriolle R. La scoliosi: suo studio tridimensionale. Milano: Ghedini, 1982.
Perricone G, Bilotta TW, Prioli L. Scoliosi e cifosi. Bologna: Istituto Ortopedico Rizzoli, 1987.
Perricone G, Bilotta TW, Prioli L. Scoliosi e cifosi. Ortesi: quando, come perché. Bologna: Istituto Ortopedico Rizzoli, 1987.
Pirola V. Cinesiologia, Milano: Edi Ermes, 1999.
Pirola V. La chinesiterapia nella rieducazione delle scoliosi. I metodi. Vol I. Milano: Sperling&Kupfer, 1993.
Pivetta M. Trattamento chinesiterapico delle scoliosi in gesso e corsetto: esercizi di routine e nuove tecniche. Le Scienze Motorie 1993; 2: 55-62.
Pivetta S. Atlante di ginnastica correttiva. Milano: Sperling&Kupfer, 1981.
Pivetta S. La tecnica della ginnastica correttiva. Scoliosi ad indicazione chirurgica, ortopedica, conservativa. Volume 2°. Milano: Sperling-&Kupfer, 1975.
Pivetta S. Le basi e la tecnica della ginnastica correttiva. Parte 1ª. Milano: Istituto Superiore di Educazione Fisica della Lombardia,1970.
Pivetta S. Le premesse della ginnastica correttiva. Milano: dispense ad uso degli studenti ISEF, 1970.
Pivetta S. Paramorfismi giovanili. Milano: Sperling-&Kupfer, 1970.
Revel M, Morin C. La reprogrammation sensorimotrice. (32° Numéro specialisè). In: Encyclopedie médico-chirurgicale Kinésitherapie Rééducation fonctionnelle. Paris: Edition Technicques, 1984.
Rigo M, Weiss HR. Il metodo Schroth nella rieducazione delle scoliosi idiopatiche: aspetti nuovi e tradizionali. Le Scienze Motorie 1993; 3: 18-31.
Rigo M, Weiss HR. Il metodo Schroth nella rieducazione delle scoliosi idiopatiche: parte 2°: i risultati. Le Scienze Motorie 1994, 1: 15-21.
Sarchi P, Fronte F, Giudici P, et al. Corsetto di Risser e adeguamento cardiorespiratorio all'esercizio muscolare. Le Scienze Motorie 1994, 1: 37-41.
Schmid C, Geiger U. Rehatrain. Esercizi di resistenza elastica. Milano: Edi.Ermes,1998.
Sibilla P, Negrini S. La valutazione del paziente scoliotico. In: Monografie Gruppo di Studio della Scoliosi. Vigevano: GSS, 1998.
Stagnara P, Charriere L. Les déviations antéro-postérieures du rachis. (11° Numéro specialisè). In: Encyclopedie médico-chirurgicale Kinésitherapie Rééducation fonctionnelle. Paris: Edition Technicques, 1977.
Stagnara P, Mollon G, De Mauroy JC. Rieducazione delle scoliosi. 2° edizione. Milano: Ghedini, 1992.
Toso B. Back School. Milano: Edi.Ermes, 2003.
Troisier O, Bilan articulaire. (44° Numéro specialisè). In: Encyclopedie médico-chirurgicale, Kinésitherapie Rééducation fonctionnelle. Paris: Edition Technicques, 1990.
Valade D, Bleton JP, Chevalier AM. Rééducation de la posture et de l'équilibre. (37° Numéro specialisè). In: Encyclopedie médico-chirurgicale, Kinésitherapie Rééducation fonctionnelle. Paris: Edition Technicques, 1987.
Various Authors. La scoliosi. Nuovi orientamenti diagnostici prognostici terapeutici. In: Atti del XX Convegno Nazionale di Chinesiologia, Vicenza 21-23 novembre 1980.
Various Authors. La scoliosi in età evolutiva: attualità e tecniche di trattamento a confronto. In: Atti del XIX Congresso G.E.K.T.S. di Modena 18-19 ottobre 1991.
Various Authors. La scoliosi, nuovi orientamenti. In: Atti del XXX Convegno Nazionale di Chinesiologia, Vicenza 1990.
Various Authors. La scoliosi. Nuovi Orientamenti diagnostici e prognostici. In: Atti del Congresso 20-21 aprile 1985. Modena 1986.
Various Authors. Le scoliosi: trattamento ortopedico lyonese nella scoliosi. Tecnica di rieducazione respiratoria nella scoliosi idiopatica grave, Firenze: Edizioni Pro Juventute,1978.
Various Authors. Scoliosi e Riabilitazione, esperienze a confronto. In: Atti del Congresso Internazio-

nale di Milano, 29-30 novembre 1985. Milano: Fondazione Pro Juventute Don Carlo Gnocchi,1985
Various Authors. Scoliosi: nuove prospettive diagnostiche e terapeutiche, Atti Convegno, Rozzano: USSL76, 1982.
Various Authors. Scoliosi. Moderne prospettive diagnostiche e terapeutiche. In: Atti del Convegno 23 ottobre 1992.
Weistein Sl. Evolutiva e conseguenze a lungo termine della scoliosi idiopatica. In: Monografie Gruppo di Studio della Scoliosi. Vigevano: GSS, 2000.
Wirhed R. Abilità atletica e anatomia del movimento. Milano: Edi.Ermes, 1986.
Xhardez Y. Vademecum del chinesiterapista, tecniche, patologia, indicazioni, Roma: Marrapese Editore, 1982.

Interview with Emanuele Rovatti

by *Federica Delucchi*

Where did your interest in scoliosis and its treatment come from, and how has your professional path developed along with the research on the topic?

Enthusiasm, curiosity, and passion have been the key words along my professional path and personal research.

The enthusiasm began when I encountered Professor Sergio Pivetta, instructor at the ISEF (Superior Institute of Physical Education) of Milan, whom I met during my studies. After encountering this first, stimulating approach, I began to immerse myself in the environment of corrective exercise with increasing curiosity and attention.

But I encountered what was perhaps the most important factor of all in the seventies and eighties, when I had the privilege of meeting a pioneering and internationally renowned figure in the specific sector of the study and treatment of scoliosis: Professor Paolo Sibilla, orthopedic specialist, vice head of the Gaetano Pini Hospital in Milan, then head of the Don Gnocchi Hospital in Milan.

Sibilla, a recognized expert in the problems of scoliosis and pathologies of the vertebral column, was a man of great passion for study, research, and spreading of knowledge; he never refused to give an opinion, to participate in a conference, to update on modern methods of study and approaches to the problems he was passionately studying – and he always did so with brilliance and enthusiasm. I followed professor Sibilla for several years, accompanying him to numerous meetings and study conferences he attended.

From the beginning of my activity in the field, I grought my patient to professor Sibilla, so much so that he himself coined the term "Rovatti's day" for those long evenings of discussion and comparison of clinical cases that I had found in my professional activity.

From those times to today, I have always followed a path of personal research, training, and growth in the various disciplines that are near to our work: ergonomics, physical kinesiotherapy, and osteopathy. Furthermore, I have had continuous experience in the field of occupational medicine.

You have always worked in the gym with your patients. What is the relationship between theory, practice, and observation?

It is truly significant to have forty years of experience. Some things are not learned from books: for me, practice, observation, and meeting with patients have all been fundamental.

Today, I follow an incredible number of cases of true vertebral pathologies and related disorders, represented in around 700 people who frequent Rovatti Plan® gyms annually. I am constantly seeing over twenty new patients a week, referred to me by colleagues, by orthopedic specialists, or simply by people I know or people who already frequent Rovatti Plan® centers.

The treatment plan is personalized for each of them. The approach always begins from a methodical and accurate postural-functional kinesiological examination, shared with the entire therapeutic team. Then the specific individual plan for treatment in the gym begins, under constant supervision.

How much time does it take to treat, improve, and/or cure a case of scoliosis? Can we have some examples of cases handled by you in relation to the patient's age and the severity of their clinical status?

Every case is different, and there are many factors that may influence the development of this type of pathology. The commitment and responsibility with which patients (often very young boys and girls) follow their medical prescriptions, therapeutic instructions, and corrective plan are key factors that should not be overlooked. Motivation also plays an important role.

If we are talking about minor scoliosis and similar conditions, I generally follow the patient for the entire period of adolescence and personal development. Very often, if the situation does not develop further toward the pathology, I advise that treatment be interrupted in order to interchange it with a sports/recreation path, which is sometimes seen as a reward for the work demonstrated by the young person.

There is no need to speak only of treatment and improvement, but also and above all of prevention of vertebral and scoliotic pathologies, which, as we know, particularly affect the White race, highly industrial societies, and those with heavy environmental pollution.

I think that if everyone had the chance at the age of puberty to better know their own vertebral column, it would be a great advantage for them in adulthood, and in many cases it could avoid or reduce the problems that generally arise.

This could be done via kinesiological postural exams, but also via scholastic itineraries with the help of a good physical education instructor and the diffusion of the proper basic knowledge on the topic, in addition to the introduction of elementary postural and ergonomic rules in daily life with the aim of avoiding back problems and true vertebral pathologies.

I have taught in schools for many years, and I am a great supporter and promoter of interaction between physical education instructors of secondary schools and kinesiologists.

Can structural scoliosis – that is, true dysmorphism – improve or be definitively cured?

As decades of work and thousands of patients have shown, satisfying results can be obtained even in cases of severe and very severe scoliosis – remembering, however, that scoliosis cannot be eliminated, and that the objective of our work is rather to obtain, over the years, a good aesthetic aspect, control of pain, and above all proper functionality of the spine such that the person not be hindered in the performance of certain activities or professions.

The results are often in relation to the perseverance and commitment of the patient. These factors are as important as a rigorous and scientific methodology in the construction and constant verification of the therapeutic protocol.

At times, when dealing primarily with young and adolescent patients, with all of the problems associated with this particular age of personal development, a bit of cooperation and a good relationship with the patient helps greatly.

Young people should be given confidence in regards to the results that they can obtain with their own effort. Collective work in the gym is also very important for this, even if each person follows a different plan. The comparison and sharing of problems are fundamental.

The final aim of the work is that patients at 18-20 years of age (that is, at the end of treatment and with their physical development completed) may have a good aesthetic aspect, at times with the improvement of the scoliotic curve, and at times with its simply not having worsened. At full skeletal maturity, good aesthetic aspect is evaluated, for example, with the improvement of the waist triangle and the improvement of the physiological curves. Above all, it is important that it be made possible for the patient to grow into an adult without pain that could adversely affect their professional development or self-esteem.

How many cases have you treated in your professional activity? What are the percentages of success?

In forty years of activity, I have seen thousands of cases. I have worked with small children, adolescents, and adults, the majority of these for many years, or at least for the entire developmental period up to adulthood. Many adults stay in treatment for ten or twenty years to continue the personalized exercises prescribed to them. The majority of cases of scoliotic pathology are followed for an average time from Risser 0 to Risser 5+; in other words, the entire pre-pubescent phase and the phase of the completion of development.

Not all of the persons I have seen have suffered from true pathologies; however, I can confirm that I have covered the entire panorama of scoliotic pathology: cases before and after surgery, many young people followed in preparation for an orthopedic corset, and then during the phase of the maintenance of the corset itself (which sometimes last several years), and finally to the removal of the corset. When there is nothing to be done and scoliosis is progressive and shows no results, neither with gym-based work nor with the orthopedic corset, casts and possibly surgery are required. I have worked with many patients during this delicate phase as well, which often requires three consecutive casts, worn for four months each (here, too, there are many schools of thought). This is, of course, a therapy that brings many difficulties for young patients, both psychologically and physically, because the musculature must be supported and strengthened during the cast phase, and these young patients must be helped in facing a difficult path.

When significant aggravation of a condition predicts a severe cardio-respiratory situation or a bad social life, surgery may be used, with evident functional and aesthetic improvements.

In 2011, I saw an excellent reduction performed at the Gaetano Pini hospital in Milan; the surgical reduction brought the scoliosis from 65-70 degrees to 19 degrees. Congratulations to the therapeutic team, but such a striking event, confirmed by the orthopedic doctors themselves, was also made possible due to good kinesiotherapeutic preparation performed for about a year leading up to the operation.

There are good results with many adult patients affected by scoliosis of around 45-50 degrees and humps greater than 20 mm in size, with normal physiological life situations. Many people obtain good and excellent results solely with corrective exercise done with extreme consistency for years, with twice-weekly appointments for corrective exercise and maintenance. Patients feel good during the routine: this, too, is a result to be emphasized, the manner in which physical and corrective exercises become positively viewed as a part of people's daily lives.

There are patients who return as adults after having followed a therapeutic plan since childhood, because they remember the well-being obtained with the consistency of the exercises.

Currently, I see about 50 patients with orthopedic corsets.

What results have you seen in your interaction with patients?

Almost all of the patients I have seen have experienced positive progress in all senses: psychological as well as physiological. Obviously, there are also, as in all cases, exceptions.

The objective data and data related to the therapeutic plan of each of the thousands of patients I have treated are all collected and ordered in an archive that is currently undergoing digitalization, because after so much time and so much experimental research, it has become necessary to make this data available for scientific research in an objectively organized manner according to precise parameters. The first exact statistical data – average success rates, percentages of healing, abandonment of work assigned, or, contrarily, of perseverance in frequenting the gym and doing the exercises according to their own personalized program – that emerge are incredibly interesting and encouraging, and first and foremost confirm the suitability of the path taken.

I remember many years ago, when I was invited to my first conferences in the early eighties, I spoke of my method, insisting on the key concept of "gaining awareness". Though my method had already been experimented with for years, I still experienced a sort of difficulty in affirming that I had obtained results that were concrete and repeatable, thus not coincidental but attributable to the method itself. Today, this is demonstrated by the numbers and the statistical data that emerge from the research and analysis of hundreds of medical records.

In contrast to the muscular biomechanical approach used in the early seventies when it was thought that the problem of scoliosis was muscular, and which was still widespread in the early eighties, I used a cortical approach following the intuitions of Sibilla and the Lyon school; that is, one based on the principal that the brain controls everything, and thus, new, correct postural information could be taught to the brain and internalized by patients.

I was very meticulous in those times, and thanks to that passion, I moved forward following these intuitions. I was thus early with the cortical-type approach, working on gaining consciousness, but without knowing it rationally.

The fact that I was meticulous and worked by touching the patient, "listening" with my hands to their body and their reactions to stimuli provided, the fact that I shared patients' situations with them: this gave me, without my wanting or meaning to have it, the chance to obtain better results than my colleagues.

It is from this, then, that your specific method was born?

Yes. I worked for years and years believing in the strength of this approach. The rest is the approach of the French school – the Lyon method – which I share fully as a philosophy. The French school applies gymnastics in a manner aimed at kyphotizing, lateralizing, and derotating the spine, but vis-a-vis, with a one-to-one relationship between patient and therapist, due to the need of physical contact between the hands of the therapist and the patient.

Moving forward into research and experimentation in the gym, I brought the method that now carries my name up-to-date. This method works partly by deepening the patient-therapist relationship until working on the development of a true relationship of empathy, and partly by overcoming the need for a one-to-one relationship that strongly limits patients' chances for accessing the therapy, also due to the elevated costs that it imposes.

With the implementation of the method of treatment with elastic bands and its continuous refinement due to collaboration with my son Marco, I have worked to make the patient ever more involved and conscious of the work to be carried out. Now we succeed in seeing more patients simultaneously, up to 10-12 persons, maintaining a personal relationship with each of them and following the individual protocol for each. One factor that I believe to be successful is the implementation of a serious corrective program, not one that is standardized, with good psychological motivation on the patient's part.

Each of my patients is seen by the entire therapeutic team at least semiannually: an appointment during which the kinesiological examination is repeated and all objective data is newly collected in order to be able to compare it with previous data.

Another cardinal point of my method is the continuous and constant sharing of progress and results collected with the entire therapeutic team that I have constructed over the years. And this happens case-by-case, person-by-person.

What have been your greatest sources of satisfaction during your career?

The results obtained over all of the years and the continuous positive results that I see every day in my patients are definitely the biggest source of satisfaction.

The recognition of students, including those who are instructors in middle and middle-high schools is another source of great satisfaction. One colleague, now a physical education instructor at a scientific high school in the province of Milan, affirmed: "You have injected your enthusiasm into my veins, and I have been bringing it to school for years". To spread passion and enthusiasm to younger colleagues is yet another source of satisfaction for me.

There are also the parents of the children I have treated, who write letters of appreciation; there are children I've treated who return after many years to follow a personalized protocol and who have positive memories of the experiences we shared. I can recount some cases of three generations of a family who returned! There are people who send their own children; there are family and orthopedic doctors who at times I barely know personally who send their patients to me because they know my method and the results obtained.

What would you wish for your younger colleagues who are facing the world of this work?

Never give in; always follow your own path with passion and enthusiasm. Never stop seeking, studying, learning. Study and training have constantly characterized my path of personal and professional growth.

At times I have learned things from young people who came to me to learn my work.

I remember, for example, a young collaborator who came from the United States for stage experience. This was in the late seventies, early eighties. She brought with her the elastic band that she used to do aerobic exercise. Seeing how she used it, I had the intuition that it could be used for the therapeutic exercises I was developing: kinesiotherapy with elastic bands for the treatment of idiopathic scoliosis.

Your exercises and trademarks carry your name: Rovatti Method® and Rovatti Plan®. How much has your professional activity, studies, and research affected your life?

Very, very much; so much that I identify with my profession, as shown in the fact that what I have done carries my name. However, I have never sacrificed my personal or family life for my work. My family has always supported me in the path of growth and research that I have decided to take, and in which I have sought to involve my family as much as possible – my children Marco and Francesca above all. My son Marco is now my greatest collaborator. But there are also other members of the Rovatti family who work with me today, who share my passion and who carry forward my ideas and the activities derived from them. The strength of family is very important to me.

In addition to them, I can speak of a very close-knit work group. The Rovatti Plan® has, today, numerous collaborators; we have strengthened the physical therapy department and the specialized branches associated with movement and rehabilitation (orthopedic technicians for insole, orthopedic specialists, and physiotherapists, to cite the principal ones). Today, we have four gyms in two specialized Rovatti Plan® centers.

Why are you only now publishing this book? And for whom?

Because of the help of my family and my great collaborators. I want, with this book, to open a path for a project that has been a dream for twenty years: to spread my method and the type of approach behind it, that of conservative treatment and multidisciplinary approach, that is team-based work. I have for many years now been illustrating this method at conventions and seminars and teaching it at specific professional development courses (among which, for example, are the national Back School courses of Professor Benedetto Toso), and at universities.

Today, I write a book that has collected all of these experiences, aimed at those working in our field. I would like this method, which has given me much satisfaction and which has been useful to hundreds, thousands of people, to be known and spread as widely as possible. I wish that it may be not only shared, but that young colleagues may bring it forward and continue research in this direction.